ENDOCRINOLOGY RESEARCH AND CLINICAL DEVELOPMENTS

TRIGLYCERIDES

CHEMICAL STRUCTURE, BIOSYNTHESIS AND ROLE IN DISEASE

Endocrinology Research and Clinical Developments

Additional books in this series can be found on Nova's website under the Series tab.

Additional e-books in this series can be found on Nova's website under the e-book tab.

Biochemistry Research Trends

Additional books in this series can be found on Nova's website under the Series tab.

Additional e-books in this series can be found on Nova's website under the e-book tab.

ENDOCRINOLOGY RESEARCH AND CLINICAL DEVELOPMENTS

TRIGLYCERIDES

CHEMICAL STRUCTURE, BIOSYNTHESIS AND ROLE IN DISEASE

CALISTA ARAUJO
AND
DEMETRIO PEREZ
EDITORS

New York

For permission to use material from this book please contact us:
Telephone 631-231-7269; Fax 631-231-8175
Web Site: http://www.novapublishers.com

Additional color graphics may be available in the e-book version of this book.

Library of Congress Cataloging-in-Publication Data

Library of Congress Control Number: 2012955266
ISBN: 978-1-62417-727-9

Published by Nova Science Publishers, Inc. † New York

CONTENTS

PREFACE

In this book, the authors discuss the chemical structure, biosynthesis and role in disease of triglycerides. Topics include lipid levels in neuropsychiatric disorders; the role of circadian clocks in the absorption and metabolism of dietary triglycerides; serum lipoprotein lipase mass as a novel biomarker of insulin sensitivity; and the effect of plasma lipids and APOE genotype on cognitive decline.

Chapter 1 - Lipids are essential components of the membranes of neurons and astrocytes and play an important role in the development and regulation of synaptic function and plasticity. Lipids regulate physical and electrical properties of neuronal cell membranes, including expression and function of membrane-associated proteins (transporters, receptors), which are targets for neuropsychotropic drugs. A number of studies suggested that various neuropsychiatric disorders and different treatment response in neuropsychiatric patients might be associated with altered brain and serum lipid levels. Since these findings are inconsistent and often contradictory, the role of lipids in the etiology and treatment of neuropsychiatric disorders is still unclear.

Some data imply that the aberration of lipid homeostasis could be the risk factor for Alzheimer's disease (AD). Lower serum lipids i.e. triglycerides (TG), total cholesterol, high-density-lipoprotein cholesterol (HDL-C) and low-density-lipoprotein cholesterol (LDL-C) levels were found in patients with AD than in healthy elderly subjects. The association between low serum cholesterol and LDL-C levels and cognitive decline during the progress of AD suggests that increased lipid levels could play the protective role in develop of AD.

The pathophysiology of mental disorders might be also related to alterations in lipid levels. Lower HDL-C values were found in patients in depressive and manic phase of bipolar disorder (BP) and major depression (MDD), and lower cholesterol levels were found in suicidal psychotic patients, while higher TG levels were found in patients with BP than in control subjects. The results imply that altered atherogenic index (cholesterol/HDL-C and LDL-C/HDL-C ratios) and inverse relationship between HDL-C and TG levels could be the hallmark of affective disorders, while lower cholesterol levels are related to suicidal behavior. The altered lipid profile suggests also that patients with BP and MDD are at higher risk for the development of coronary heart disease.

Lipids are shown to interact with serotonergic system, while mental disorders have been connected to alterations in both, serotonergic and lipid system. It has been shown that the increase in platelet serotonin concentrations and decrease in serum cholesterol and LDL-C levels could be the characteristic features of psychotic subtype in patients in a manic phase of BP.

The effects of serotonin are regulated by several types of its receptors. Pharmacological and genetic research suggest the relationship between lipid profile and serotonergic type 1B (5-HT1B), 2A (5-HT2A) and 2C (5-HT2C) receptors. In agreement, serum cholesterol levels were associated with 5-HT1B receptor gene polymorphism in healthy subjects.

The data on the association between the treatment response to antidepressants and lipid profile are scarce and inconsistent. It has been shown that this relationship depends of the structural and functional characteristics of antidepressant dugs. Baseline total cholesterol, TG and LDL-C levels were higher in nonresponders than in responders to paroxetine (selective serotonin reuptake inhibitor), but not to tianeptine (serotonin reuptake enhancer) acute treatment in non-suicidal patients with MDD.

Further studies are needed to confirm and extend the findings that altered lipid profile could play a significant role in the pathogenesis, progress and treatment response in various neuropsychiatric disorders.

Chapter 2 - Hyperlipidemia is a major risk factor for cardiovascular disease. And there is evidence to suggest that plasma lipids exhibit diurnal variations. Light is known to affect diurnal variations by entraining cells in the suprachiasmatic nucleus (SCN) of the hypothalamus region of the brain. Within these cells, positive and negative transcriptional feedback loops constitute a molecular Clock in mammals. Two transcription factors, Clock and Bmal1, play critical role in determining the circadian variations. Recent studies reveal that molecular components of the Clock system are not only in the SCN but also found within the cells of peripheral tissues, such as the gastrointestinal tract and liver. Mutant Clock gene mice are obese and show hypertriglyceridemia.

Triglyceride are the chemical form in which more than 90% of dietary fat are hydrolyzed in the intestinal lumen to free fatty acids and monoacylglycerols, which are taken up and resynthesized into triglyceride in enterocytes. Triglyceride homeostasis in the body is mainly controlled by endogenous synthesis, intestinal absorption, and hepatic metabolism. Intestinal lipid absorption and metabolism is an essential physiological process that is regulated by Clock.

This Chapter describes the molecular mechanisms that co-ordinate the absorption of triglyceride from the diet and its release into the circulation by an overview of liver cellular triglyceride metabolism and intestinal absorption regulation, as well as the function of key proteins involved in these processes, with particular emphasis on the Clock's role in triglyceride homeostasis, as it is the main target of triglyceride deposition in pathological hypertriglyceridemia. Current knowledge on Clock's role in maintaining triglyceride homeostasis and how their dysregulation leads to the pathogenesis of obesity are discussed. Future work in this area will provide a clearer picture regarding the regulation of intestinal lipid absorption and liver fat metabolism by circadian Clocks.

Chapter 3 - Lipoprotein lipase (LPL) plays an important role in the absorption of TG from the bloodstream into the tissues. LPL abnormalities cause hypertriglyceridemia and low high-density lipoprotein (HDL)-cholesterol levels. LPL mass is usually measured after a heparin injection (postheparin LPL mass). LPL mass was found to exist in the serum before heparin injection (preheparin serum). The preheparin LPL mass is not active, and the role of this serum LPL mass is not known. The authors sought to clarify the role of LPL. The administration of troglitazone, an insulin-sensitizer, increased the serum LPL mass, as did an insulin injection. Metabolic syndrome severity is negatively related to serum LPL mass. The homeostasis model assessment of insulin resistance (HOMA-IR) is also correlated with serum LPL mass. These data suggest that the LPL mass reflects the LPL production in the entire body and might be a good marker of insulin sensitivity.

Working from this assumption, the authors have assessed the effects of various lipid- and glucose-targeting drugs on LPL mass and have found several interesting results.

1. Metformin, which is mainly thought to reduce glucose synthesis in the liver, increased the serum LPL mass in type 2 diabetes mellitus patients. Thus, the authors observed a previously unidentified effect of metformin. In an in vitro study, metformin enhanced the LPL produced by skeletal muscle cells through the activation of adenosine monophosphate-activated protein kinase (AMPK); however, this effect was not observed in adipocytes.
2. 3-hydroxy-3-methylglutaryl coenzyme A (HMG-CoA) reductase inhibitors (statins) are widely used to reduce serum low-density lipoprotein cholesterol (LDL-C) levels. Some statins reduce serum TG levels and increase serum high-density lipoprotein cholesterol (HDL-C) levels. Pravastatin and atorvastatin increase preheparin LPL mass in patients with type 2 diabetes. Simvastatin and pitavastatin increase LPL activity in adipocytes. In skeletal muscle cells, atorvastatin and pitavastatin enhance LPL production through the activation of AMPK.

This review will define serum LPL mass and describe the effects of several lipid- and glucose-targeting drugs on serum LPL mass, in addition to discussing new mechanisms regulating triglyceride metabolism in adipocytes and skeletal muscle cells.

Chapter 4 - Although the presence of an APOE4 allele increases the risk of Alzheimer's disease (AD), there is no current evidence that the cognitive decline among those with an APOE4 allele can be prevented. Detrimental effects of APOE4 may be exacerbated by synergistic preventable risk factors, such as plasma lipids. The authors therefore examined the combined effect of plasma lipids and APOE genotype on cognitive function in elderly individuals. Plasma concentrations of high-density lipoprotein (HDL), low-density lipoprotein (LDL), triglyceride (TG), total cholesterol (TC), apolipoprotein E (apoE) were evaluated in 622 community-dwelling individuals aged 65 years and older. The authors investigated the associations between plasma lipids and cognitive function in APOE4 carrier (E4+) and APOE4 non-carrier (E4-) groups using 3-year longitudinal data. At baseline and 3 years later, cognitive scores were correlated with plasma apoE levels in both E4- and E4+, and HDL level in E4-. The authors' findings suggest that an interaction between apoE and HDL is affected by APOE4, and is possibly linked with a protective effect on cognitive decline in later life. Preservation of higher plasma apoE and HDL from early life is proposed as a possible strategy for maintaining cognitive function in later life, especially for APOE4-positive individuals.

In: Triglycerides
Editors: C. Araujo and D. Perez
ISBN: 978-1-62417-727-9

Chapter 1

LIPID LEVELS IN NEUROPSYCHIATRIC DISORDERS

Dubravka Svob Strac[1], Maja Mustapic[1], Marina Sagud[2], Suzana Uzun[3], Oliver Kozumplik[3], Paola Presecki[4], Matea Nikolac[1], Ninoslav Mimica[3], Gordana Nedic[1], Alma Mihaljevic Peles[2], Mladen Pavlovic[5], Darko Marcinko[2], Nela Pivac[1] and Dorotea Muck-Seler[1,*]

[1]Rudjer Boskovic Institute, Division of Molecular Medicine, Zagreb, Croatia
[2]University Hospital Center Zagreb, Clinic for Psychiatry, Zagreb, Croatia
[3]Clinics for Psychiatry Vrapce, Zagreb, Croatia
[4]Psychiatric Hospital Sveti Ivan, Jankomir, Zagreb, Croatia
[5]Institute for Medical Research and Occupational Health, Zagreb, Croatia

[*] Corresponding author: Dorotea Muck-Seler, Ph.D., Senior Scientist. Rudjer Boskovic Institute, Division of Molecular Medicine, Bijenicka cesta 54, 10 000 Zagreb, Croatia. Phone: 385 1 457 1207, Fax: + 385 1 456 1010. E-mail: seler@irb.hr.

ABSTRACT

Lipids are essential components of the membranes of neurons and astrocytes and play an important role in the development and regulation of synaptic function and plasticity. Lipids regulate physical and electrical properties of neuronal cell membranes, including expression and function of membrane-associated proteins (transporters, receptors), which are targets for neuropsychotropic drugs. A number of studies suggested that various neuropsychiatric disorders and different treatment response in neuropsychiatric patients might be associated with altered brain and serum lipid levels. Since these findings are inconsistent and often contradictory, the role of lipids in the etiology and treatment of neuropsychiatric disorders is still unclear.

Some data imply that the aberration of lipid homeostasis could be the risk factor for Alzheimer's disease (AD). Lower serum lipids i.e. triglycerides (TG), total cholesterol, high-density-lipoprotein cholesterol (HDL-C) and low-density-lipoprotein cholesterol (LDL-C) levels were found in patients with AD than in healthy elderly subjects. The association between low serum cholesterol and LDL-C levels and cognitive decline during the progress of AD suggests that increased lipid levels could play the protective role in develop of AD.

The pathophysiology of mental disorders might be also related to alterations in lipid levels. Lower HDL-C values were found in patients in depressive and manic phase of bipolar disorder (BP) and major depression (MDD), and lower cholesterol levels were found in suicidal psychotic patients, while higher TG levels were found in patients with BP than in control subjects. The results imply that altered atherogenic index (cholesterol/HDL-C and LDL-C/HDL-C ratios) and inverse relationship between HDL-C and TG levels could be the hallmark of affective disorders, while lower cholesterol levels are related to suicidal behavior. The altered lipid profile suggests also that patients with BP and MDD are at higher risk for the development of coronary heart disease.

Lipids are shown to interact with serotonergic system, while mental disorders have been connected to alterations in both, serotonergic and lipid system. It has been shown that the increase in platelet serotonin concentrations and decrease in serum cholesterol and LDL-C levels could be the characteristic features of psychotic subtype in patients in a manic phase of BP.

The effects of serotonin are regulated by several types of its receptors. Pharmacological and genetic research suggest the relationship between lipid profile and serotonergic type 1B (5-HT1B), 2A (5-HT2A) and 2C (5-HT2C) receptors. In agreement, serum cholesterol levels were associated with 5-HT1B receptor gene polymorphism in healthy subjects.

The data on the association between the treatment response to antidepressants and lipid profile are scarce and inconsistent. It has been shown that this relationship depends of the structural and functional characteristics of antidepressant dugs. Baseline total cholesterol, TG and LDL-C levels were higher in nonresponders than in responders to paroxetine (selective serotonin reuptake inhibitor), but not to tianeptine (serotonin reuptake enhancer) acute treatment in non-suicidal patients with MDD.

Further studies are needed to confirm and extend the findings that altered lipid profile could play a significant role in the pathogenesis, progress and treatment response in various neuropsychiatric disorders.

1. Lipids and the Central Nervous System

Lipids are important structural components of the cell membranes that provide not only a permeability barrier, but also an environment essential for the proper functioning of different membrane-bound proteins [Maxfield and Tabas, 2005]. Namely, lipids regulate thickness and permeability/fluidity of cell membranes by which they can influence not only trans-membrane exchange, but also the function of membrane-associated proteins. Lipids are demonstrated to have a role in enzyme function, regulation of receptor expression, and they also serve as precursors for various second messengers [Adibhatla and Hatcher, 2008]. In that way, they are involved in many important biological functions of the cells, including cellular adhesion [Hakomori, 2002], permeability to toxins and pathogen attachment [Taïeb et al., 2004], signal transduction [Berridge, 1984; Fantini and Barrantes, 2009], and protein trafficking [Anderson and Jacobson, 2002]. Moreover, as a part of mitochondrial membranes, lipids are necessary for function of the mitochondrial respiratory chain and oxidative phosphorylation, influencing energy production [Adibhatla and Hatcher, 2008].

Lipid metabolism is of particular importance for the central nervous system (CNS), which contains the highest concentration of lipids next to adipose tissue [Adibhatla and Hatcher, 2008]. Lipids, and within particularly the cholesterol, are the essential components of the myelin sheath and the membranes of neurons and astrocytes. They play a crucial role in the development and regulation of synaptic function and plasticity by ensuring the proper fidelity and timing of signal transmission. Namely, as an essential part of the neuronal cell membrane, lipids regulate electrical properties of the membrane and expression of proteins, such as neurotransmitter receptors and transporters, embedded in the membrane lipid bilayer. Moreover, cholesterol is the precursor in the synthesis of steroid hormones, which serve both peripheral and central communication functions [Hu et al., 2010], as well as of neurosteroids, which promote neurogenesis and modulate neurotransmission [Karishma and Herbert, 2002; Suzuki et al., 2004; Wang et al., 2005].

Hence, by influencing conformation, function and trafficking of neurotransmitter receptors and transporters, enzymes and second messengers, optimal lipid levels are important for their normal functioning and availability [Burger and Gimpl, 2000; Fantini and Barrantes, 2009; Baier and Barrantes, 2007; Allen et al., 2007]. Gamma-aminobutyric acid (GABA), serotonin, and glutamate, as well as peptidic neurotransmitters such as leucine enkephalin, alpha-melanocyte stimulating hormone (MSH) and substance P, have been reported to interact with lipids present on neural cell membranes [Allen et al., 2007; Fantini and Barrantes, 2009]. As indispensable partners of these various neurotransmitter effector systems, lipids have been implicated in major neural functions including brain development, neuritogenesis, memory formation, synaptic transmission, and aging [Ichikawa et al., 2009; Gorio et al., 1986; Fantini and Barrantes, 2009].

The crucial role of lipids in the brain physiology is also demonstrated by many different neurological and psychiatric disorders, including major depression, bipolar disorder, schizophrenia, altered behaviors such as suicidal behavior [Marcinko et al., 2011], and neurodegenerative diseases such as Alzheimer's and Parkinson's disease, that involve deregulated lipid metabolism [Adibhatla and Hatcher, 2007]. Moreover, different treatment response in neuropsychiatric patients might be associated with altered brain and serum lipid levels, as they may affect targets for numerous neuropsychotropic drugs. These findings are inconsistent and often contradictory and consequently the role of lipids in the etiology and treatment of neuropsychiatric disorders is still unclear. Better understanding of the lipid metabolism in various CNS disorders could open the opportunities for development of new drugs and therapies.

2. Lipids in Alzheimer's Disease

In addition to two biochemical hallmarks of Alzheimer's disease, gathering of amyloid-beta peptides (Aß) in senile plaques and accumulation of hyperphosphorylated protein tau in neurofibrillary tangles [Koudinov and Koudinova, 2005], a variety of potential biomarkers for this progressive neurodegenerative disorder has been widely investigated, including biomarkers of lipoprotein metabolism as well [Solfrizzi et al., 2006; Song et al., 2009]. Despite the intensive research of the lipid role in the development and progression of Alzheimer's disease [Adibhatla and Hatcher, 2008], results are confusing and often contradictory [Panza et al., 2006]. Some studies have demonstrated that high lipid levels may be associated with increased [Kuo et al., 1998; Notkola et al., 1998; Cagnin et al., 2007] or decreased [Reitz et al., 2004, Mielke et al., 2005] risk for Alzheimer's disease, while the others [Tan et al., 2003] have found no relationship between lipid levels and development of Alzheimer's disease.

Various studies investigated the association between cholesterol levels, amyloid precursor protein (APP) metabolism and apolipoprotein E (ApoE) phenotype [Chauhan, 2003; Michikawa, 2003]. ApoE is one of the major apolipoproteins in plasma and the principal cholesterol carrier protein in the brain. The finding that possession of the ε4 allele of ApoE gene presents a significant risk factor for Alzheimer's disease provided strong evidence for a role of cholesterol in the pathogenesis of this disease [Puglielli, 2008]. Some authors also demonstrated that cholesterol homeostasis in the brain might influence the expression of the APP and Aß in patients with Alzheimer's disease [Koudinov and Koudinova, 2005; Shobab, 2005; Canevari and Clark, 2007]. Elevated brain cholesterol levels have been shown to increase the formation and deposition of Aß plaques from APP in vitro and in vivo models, while drugs such as statins that inhibit cholesterol synthesis lower Aß levels [Hartmann et al., 2007; Puglielli, 2008; Whitfield, 2006]. Although decreased prevalence of Alzheimer's disease could be associated with the use of statins [Wolozin et al., 2000; Jick et al., 2000; Caballero and Nahata, 2004], this may be due to their well-known antioxidant and anti-inflammatory properties [Jick et al., 2000], rather then to their cholesterol-lowering effects.

In contrast to the reports showing higher [Ramdane and Daoudi-Gueddah, 2011], lower [Solfrizzi et al., 2006; Reitz et al., 2004], or unaltered [Kuo et al., 1998] total serum cholesterol levels in patients with Alzheimer's disease compared to healthy elderly subjects, most literature data suggest no alteration in serum triglyceride (TG) levels in Alzheimer's disease [Kuo et al., 1998; Mielke et al., 2005; Merched et al., 2000]. Moreover, some authors reported that high total cholesterol is a risk factor for dementia in midlife, but not in late-life, while high total cholesterol in late-life may be an indicator of better health status [Panza et al., 2006]. In addition, lower high-density lipoprotein cholesterol (HDL-C) levels in patients with Alzheimer's disease compared to healthy elderly subjects were found in some [Kuo et al., 1998; Merched et al.,

2000] but not in all [Reitz et al., 2004] studies. Some authors suggested that high HDL-C levels in elderly individuals may be associated with a decreased risk of Alzheimer's disease [Reitz et al., 2010]. The lower amounts of neurosteroids, such as pregnenolone and dehydroepiandrosterone, for whose biosynthesis cholesterol is essential, have been observed in the brains of patients with Alzheimer's disease in correlation with increased levels of Aß and phosphorylated tau proteins. Considering neuroprotective properties of many neurosteroids, their lower levels may contribute to Aß neurotoxicity [Wang et al., 2007].

Studies demonstrating elevated lipid peroxidation in Alzheimer's disease support a role of oxidative damage in this disorder, indicating that lipid peroxidation occurs early in the development of Alzheimer's disease [Williams et al., 2006]. The membrane levels of ethanolamine plasmalogen, which constitutes membrane structures and regulates cholesterol transport and signaling, were significantly decreased in the neurons of the cortex and hippocampus [Kawarabayashi and Shoji, 2008], as well as in serum of patients with Alzheimer's disease [Goodenowe et al., 2007], while the extent of this decrease correlated with the severity of dementia.

2.1. Subjects and Methods

Subjects

The study included 50 female patients with Alzheimer's disease and 58 age-matched healthy older females recruited from the local senior centers [Presecki et al., 2011]. All participants or their guardians gave informed consent. The study was performed in accordance with the ethical standards laid down in the 1964 Declaration of Helsinki and was approved by the local Ethics Committee.

All patients with Alzheimer's disease met the diagnostic criteria of the probable Alzheimer's disease according to the Diagnostic and Statistical Manual of Mental Disorders, fourth edition (DSM-IV) [American Psychiatric Association, 2000] and the criteria of the National Institute of Neurological and Communicative Disorders and Stroke and the Alzheimer's Disease and Related Disorders Association (NINDS-ADRDA) [McKhann et al., 1984]. The exclusion criteria for all patients were the diagnoses of severe somatic diseases, major functional psychiatric disorders, smoking, alcoholism and use of cholesterol-lowering drugs.

Cognitive impairment was evaluated using Mini Mental State Examination (MMSE) [Folstein et al., 1975] that was translated and validated to Croatian population (www.parinc.com). Patients were subdivided according to the MMSE scores into two groups: patients in the middle stage of Alzheimer's disease with MMSE scores 15.1 ± 3.5 (range 10–17) and patients in the late stage of AD with MMSE scores 1.6 ± 2.4 (range 0–9). In the group of patients with Alzheimer's disease subdivided according to the different phases of the disease, patients in the late phase of Alzheimer's disease were significantly ($p < 0.008$, Tukey's test following ANOVA) older then the patients in the middle phase of the disease. There was a significant negative correlation (r = –0.345, $p = 0.0142$) between MMSE scores and age of patients with Alzheimer's disease.

Psychotic features were evaluated by means of the Neuropsychiatric Inventory [Cummings et al., 1994] and the patients with Alzheimer's disease were subdivided according to the presence of psychotic (MMSE scores 8 ± 7.5, range 0–16) or non-psychotic features (MMSE scores 6.1 ± 7.1, range 0–17). The subjects in the control group had MMSE scores from 27 to 30 (28.7 ± 1.2). As expected, a significant ($p < 0.001$, ANOVA) difference in the severity of dementia was observed between patients with Alzheimer's disease (MSSE scores = 6.8 ± 7.2) and healthy controls (MSSE scores = 28.7 ± 1.2). There were also significant differences in MMSE scores within the group of patients with Alzheimer's disease ($p < 0.001$), where patients in the middle phase of Alzheimer's disease had higher (15.1 ± 3.5), while patients in the late phase of Alzheimer's disease had lower (1.6 ± 2.4) MMSE scores.

Patients with Alzheimer's disease were still significantly ($p < 0.001$) older then control subjects. The healthy controls had lipid levels within normal range and they were evaluated with a clinical interview to rule out for Axis I disorders, current and past medical status and MMSE. Exclusion criteria were the use of cholesterol-lowering drugs, smoking and alcoholism. The number and the age of healthy subjects and patients with Alzheimer's disease, subdivided in different groups, are listed in Table 1.

Methods

Serum cholesterol, HDL-C and TG levels were determined by the enzymatic color test for clinical analyzers, with the linearity within concentrations range of 0.64–18 mmol/L for cholesterol, 0.05–4.65 mmol/L for HDL-C and 0.11–11.40 mmol/L for TG. Serum LDL-C levels were determined by the enzymatic clearance assay, with linearity up to 22.4 mmol/L.

Table 1. The number and the age of healthy controls and patients with Alzheimer's disease (AD), subdivided in different groups

Subjects	N	Age/Mean ± SD (range)
Healthy controls	58	71.6 ± 6.2 (63–90)
All patients with AD	50	79.1 ± 9.0 (56-96)
Patients with middle stage of AD	19	74.8 ± 9.9 (56-89)
Patients with late stage of AD	31	81.7 ± 4.5 (57–96)
AD patients with psychotic features	13	76.0 ± 11.6 (56-96)
AD patients without psychotic features	37	80.1 ± 7.8 (57–94)

Statistical Analysis

All data are presented as Mean ± SD. Statistical analyses were performed with SigmaStat 3.1 (Jandell Scientific Corp., San Raphael, California, USA). The differences between groups were assessed by one-way analysis of variance (ANOVA), followed by Tukey's test. The correlations between MMSE scores, age and lipid values were determined by a Pearson's coefficient of correlation. The results were considered significant when $p < 0.05$.

2.2. Results

Our results demonstrated that all patients with Alzheimer's disease had lower serum cholesterol ($F_{1,106} = 5.54$, $p < 0.020$), TG ($F_{1,106} = 4.945$, $p < 0.028$), LDL-C ($F_{1,106} = 4.7814$, $p < 0.031$) and HDL-C ($F_{1,106} = 6.861$ $p < 0.010$) levels then healthy controls (Figure 1). Moreover, the levels of serum cholesterol ($F_{1,105} = 6.342$, $p = 0.003$), TG ($F_{1,105} = 3.473$, $p < 0.035$), LDL-C ($F_{1,105} = 5.272$, $p = 0.007$) and HDL-C ($F_{1,105} = 3.779$, $p = 0.026$) were also significantly different between patients in various stages of the disease and healthy subjects.

Namely, as shown in the Table 2, patients in the late stage of Alzheimer's disease had significantly lower levels of serum cholesterol, TG, HDL-C and LDL-C then healthy subjects, as well as significantly lower levels of cholesterol, and LDL-C then patients in the middle stage of the disease. Serum cholesterol ($p < 0.044$), HDL-C ($p = 0.037$) and LDL-C ($p < 0.037$) levels also differed among psychotic and non-psychotic patients and healthy controls. Significantly lower serum cholesterol, HDL-C and LDL-C levels were observed in patients with non-psychotic features than in healthy subjects, while TG levels were not significantly different among analyzed groups (Figure 1). No significant differences in serum lipid levels were observed between patients with Alzheimer's disease subdivided according to the presence of psychotic features.

Table 2. Serum lipid levels in healthy controls and in patients with Alzheimer's disease (AD) in the middle and late stage of the disease

	Healthy controls (58)	Patients with AD (50)	
		Middle stage (19)	Late stage (31)
Cholesterol (mmol/L)	5.70 ± 1.29	5.71 ± 1.08	4.79 ± 1.11* #
HDL-C (mmol/L)	1.71 ± 0.46	1.57 ± 0.39	1.46 ± 0.37*
LDL-C (mmol/L)	3.45 ± 0.97	3.43 ± 0.93	2.79 ± 0.95* #
TG (mmol/L)	1.66 ± 0.99	1.50 ± 0.78	1.16 ± 0.56*

* $p < 0.02$, $p < 0.01$ vs. healthy controls, # $p < 0.049$ vs. patients in the middle stage of AD.

Our results demonstrated the significant correlation between MMSE scores and serum cholesterol (r = 0.348, $p = 0.013$) and LDL-C (r = 0.302, $p < 0.033$) levels, but not between MMSE scores and serum HDL-C (r = 0.165, $p = 0.251$) and TG (r = 0.174, $p = 0.236$) levels in patients with Alzheimer's disease. There was no significant correlation of age with cholesterol, HDL-C, LDL-C and TG levels in healthy controls and in patients with Alzheimer's disease.

3. Lipids and Mood Disorders

Various reports have suggested that alterations in the lipid profile may pay a role in the pathophysiology of mood disorders; however, they yielded very inconsistent results. Previous studies have indicated that patients diagnosed with major depressive disorder (MDD) may have significantly different lipid levels compared to healthy subjects [Fava et al., 1996]. Although some studies demonstrated elevated cholesterol levels in subjects with major depression [Bajwa et al., 1992; Weider et al., 1992; Nakao et al., 2001; Nakao and Jano, 2004], some authors found no relationship between cholesterol and depression

[Freedman et al., 1995; McCallum et al., 1994; Oxenkrug et al., 1983; Huang, 2005; Shibata et al., 1999; Brown et al., 1994]. However, the majority of reports suggested that major depression is associated with lower serum and brain cholesterol levels [Morgan et al., 1993; Lindberg et al., 1994; Maes et al., 1994, 1997; Cadeddu et al., 1995; Olusi and Fido, 1996; Horsten et al., 1997; Suarez, 1999; Rabe-Jablonska and Poprawska, 2000; Steegmans et al., 2000; Terao et al., 2000a; Rafter, 2001; Partonen et al., 1999; Beasley et al., 2005].

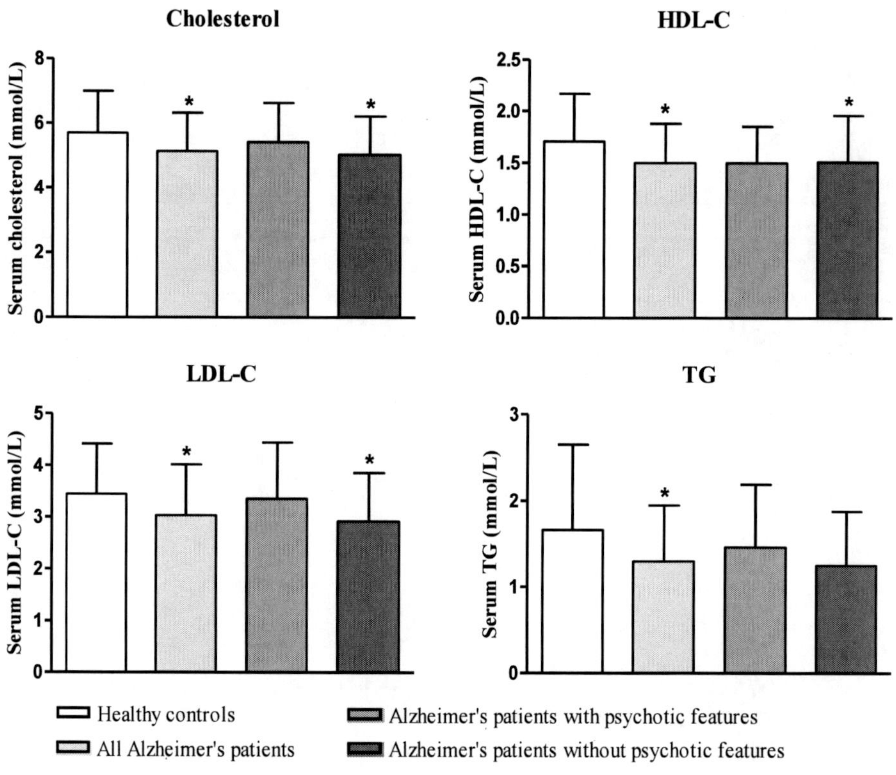

Figure 1. Serum cholesterol, high-density-lipoprotein cholesterol (HDL-C), low-density-lipoprotein cholesterol (LDL-C) and triglycerides (TG) levels in healthy controls (N = 58) and in patients with Alzheimer's disease (N= 50), subdivided according to the presence of psychotic (N = 13) or non-psychotic features (N = 37). Results are expressed as means ± SD. $*p < 0.05$ vs. corresponding values in the healthy controls (ANOVA following Tukey's test).

Low cholesterol levels have also been found to increase the risk of MDD [Partonen et al., 1999], as well the risk of suicide in depression [Rabe-Jablonska and Poprawska, 2000; Partonen et al., 1999; Sarchiapone et al., 2001], and to correlate with the severity of depressive symptoms [Rabe-Jablonska and Poprawska, 2000; Rafter, 2001; Steegmans et al., 2000; Morgan et al., 1993; Horsten et al., 1997; Chen et al., 2001]. Low esterified cholesterol levels are also observed in relatives of depressed patients [Maes et al., 1994] suggesting possible genetic factors involved. Some studies have reported higher cholesterol levels following pharmacotherapy in patients with major depressive symptoms [Gabriel, 2007]. Furthermore, a cholesterol-lowering diet was found to result in a decrease in depressive symptoms [Weidner et al., 1992]. The increase in the activity of enzymes involved in lipid oxidation and peroxidation [Bilici et al., 2001] has been demonstrated in depressed patients.

Various data have been also presented on the entire lipid profile (i.e. cholesterol, HDL-C, LDL-C, and TG) in affective disorders. Some authors found a negative linear association of depressive symptoms with HDL-C, but not with TC levels [Horsten et al., 1997]. On the other hand, other group [Maes et al., 1997] found that both serum HDL-C and TC levels were lower in depressed patients then in control subjects. Patients with long-term depressive symptoms have been reported to have lower HDL-C values and higher pro-atherogenic indices (i.e., LDL-C/HDL-C and TC/HDL-C) then healthy subjects [Lehto et al., 2008]. Lower levels of HDL-C have been also observed in depressed macaque females [Shively et al., 2005] and in women who scored higher for depression [Chen et al., 2001]. It has been found that depression was inversely associated with TC levels and the ratio of TC to HDL-C [Suarez, 1999]. Moreover, first degree relatives of bipolar patients had lower HDL-C levels than corresponding healthy controls [Sobczak et al., 2004].

Some studies demonstrated that TC and LDL-C values were lower in men who had experienced low mood [Lindberg et al., 1994], and that they significantly related to the progression of depressive status [Shibata et al., 1999]. Low levels of TC and LDL-C in patients with acute depressive symptoms were observed, which increased significantly during the remission of depressive symptoms [Rabe-Jabłonska and Poprawska, 2000]. Correlations between TC levels and negative mood have been reported in older women [Troisi et al., 2001], while Brown et al. (2004) found increased depressive symptoms among women with naturally occurring lower levels of TC and LDL-C. On the other hand, some authors have proposed that depressive patients have lower LDL-C, but higher HDL-C and TG levels [Glueck et al.,

1994]. Other studies also suggested that patients with mood disorders are at increased risk of hypertriglyceridemia [Fiedorowicz et al., 2008].

Patients with seasonal affective disorder (SAD) had significantly lower total cholesterol levels than control subjects [Pjrek et al., 2007], and decreased cholesterol levels were also found in patients with mania [Ghaemi et al., 2000; Atmaca et al., 2002a; Cassidy and Carroll, 2002; Pae et al., 2004; Sagud et al., 2007].

In contrast to the depression, higher cholesterol levels have been demonstrated in patients with anxiety disorders including panic disorder (PD), generalized anxiety disorder (GAD), obsessive compulsive disorder (OCD) and post-traumatic stress disorder (PTSD) [Hayward et al., 1989; Bajwa et al., 1992; Kuczmierczyk et al., 1996; Agargun et al., 1998; Kagan et al., 1999; Sevincok et al., 2001; Peter et al., 2002]. Moreover, patients with co-morbid depression and anger attacks were found to have elevated cholesterol levels [Fava et al., 1996]. It has been suggested that the effects of anxiety on cholesterol might be mediated through increases in noradrenergic tone [Charney and Redmond, 1983; Villacres et al., 1987], activity of lipoprotein lipase [Hayward et al., 1989] and free fatty acids [Hayward et al., 1989]. It has also been proposed that elevated cholesterol may also directly contribute to anxiety by altering the sensitivity of the GABA receptors [Sooksawate and Simmonds, 1998; 2001]. However, in contrast to these studies some authors reported that low concentrations of TC and LDL-C might be associated with increased anxiety [Conklin and Stanford, 2008].

3.1. Lipid Levels in Affective Disorders

3.1.1. Subjects and Methods

Subjects

The study included 41 female medication-free patients diagnosed with bipolar I disorder, (22 patients (age mean ± SD, 48.5 ± 13.2) in manic and 19 patients (age mean ± SD, 44.1 ± 12.9) in depressive episodes) and 34 female patients (age mean ± SD, 50.1 ± 6.6) with major depression [Sagud et al., 2009]. The diagnoses were made by using the Structured Clinical Interview for DSM-IV disorders [American Psychiatric Association, 1994]. Manic patients scored at least 18 on the Young Mania Rating Scale (YMRS) [Young et al., 1978] and 7 or less on the 17-item Hamilton Depression Rating Scale HAMD-17 [Hamilton, 1960]. Patients with bipolar depression or major depressive disorder scored at least 18 on the HAMD-17, and 5 or less on the YMRS. Table 3 presents the clinical characteristics of the patients.

Exclusion criteria were diagnoses of schizophrenia, dementia, schizoaffective disorder, alcohol abuse in the previous month, serious medical disease (including cardiovascular disease), no change ± 5% of their body weight in the previous 3 months, elevated (> 7.0 mmol/L) cholesterol levels, use of cholesterol-lowering drugs, pregnancy, lactation and suicidal behavior (patients who scored 2 or more on item 3 on the HAMD-17). All patients had been free of psychotropic medication for at least 2 weeks before study entry, except for a benzodiazepine-equivalent dose of 2 mg of lorazepam daily.

The control group (age mean ± SD, 44.7 ± 12.8) consisted of 50 medication-free healthy female subjects, recruited mostly from medical staff, with no personal history of any psychiatric disorder. Nine patients with mania, seven patients in the depressive phase of bipolar disorder, 13 patients with major depression and 17 healthy controls were in menopause.

The body mass index (BMI) was calculated by dividing the weight (in kilograms) by squared height (in meters). The BMI for healthy controls was 24.0 ± 4.5 kg/m2, for major depressive disorder were 24.3 ± 2.2 kg/m2, while for manic and depressive episode of the bipolar disorder the BMI values were 24.7 ± 4.5 and 23.3 ± 2.4 kg/m2, respectively. No significant difference in age ($p = 0.11$, ANOVA) and BMI ($p = 0.19$) was observed between groups.

Written informed consent was obtained from all participants, and all procedures were in accordance with the Helsinki Declaration and approved by the Local Ethics Committee.

Table 3. The clinical characteristics of the patients

Data are presented as mean ± SD	Bipolar disorder		Major depressive disorder
	Manic episode	Depressive episode	
YMRS total scores	26.1 ± 6.0	-	-
HAMD total scores	5.7 ± 1.6	27.3 ± 4.2	26.1 ± 2.2
Disorder duration (years)	9.4 ± 9.6	12.5 ± 9.8	12.7 ± 10.4
Current episode duration (days)	10.4 ± 11.3	4.2 ± 3.0	3.2 ± 1.5
Number of prior manic episodes	5.2 ± 7.5	4.6 ± 5.8	-
Number of prior depressive episodes	6.7 ± 9.2	7.9 ± 7.8	3.1 ± 2.9

Methods

Serum cholesterol, HDL-C and TG levels were determined in the blood samples drawn in the morning after a 12 h overnight fast. The enzymatic color test for clinical analyzers had the linearity within concentrations in the range of 0.64–18 mmol/L, 0.05–4.65 mmol/L and 0.11–11.40 mmol/L for serum cholesterol, HDL-C and TG, respectively. Serum LDL-C levels were determined by enzymatic clearance assay, with linearity up to 22.4 mmol/L.

Statistical Analysis

The results are expressed as mean ± S.D. Statistical analysis of results was performed by SigmaStat 3.1. Data was evaluated using one-way analysis of variance (ANOVA), followed by Tukey's Honestly Significant Difference (HSD) test for multiple comparisons. Analysis of covariance (ANCOVA) was used with age, smoking and menopause as covariates. *P*-values of < 0.05 were considered significant.

3.1.2. Results

Serum TG levels were significant ($p < 0.000$) different among groups (Table 4). Namely, TG values were significantly higher in serum of patients with bipolar disorders in manic ($p = 0.007$, Tukey's HDS test) or depressive ($p < 0.001$ Tukey's HDS test) episodes than in healthy controls. Moreover, serum TG levels were significantly ($p < 0.048$) higher in bipolar disorder patients in a depressed phase than in patients with major depression. TG levels differed also significantly among groups after of adjustment of data with age ($p < 0.001$), smoking ($p < 0.000$) and menopause ($p < 0.001$) as covariates (ANCOVA).

The results also demonstrated that healthy controls and patients with major depressive or bipolar disorder had significantly ($p = 0.000$) different serum HDL-C levels (Table 4). Namely, significantly lower serum HDL-C values were observed in patients with bipolar disorder both in manic ($p < 0.001$; Tukey's HSD) or depressive ($p < 0.001$, Tukey's test) episodes, as well as with major depression ($p < 0.001$, Tukey's test), in comparison with HDL-C levels in healthy subjects. HDL-C levels also differed significantly among groups when data were adjusted with age ($p < 0.000$), smoking ($p < 0.000$) and menopause ($p < 0.000$) as covariates (ANCOVA).

In contrast, serum cholesterol and LDL-C concentrations did not differ significantly between healthy controls and patients with major depression or bipolar disorder (Figure 2). Age ($p = 0.218$; $p = 0.089$), smoking status ($p = 0.811$; $p = 0.226$) and menopause ($p = 0.746$; $p = 0.224$) of the subjects had no significant effect on serum cholesterol and LDL-C levels, respectively

(ANCOVA). As shown in Figure 2, the atherogenic index was significantly different among groups. Namely, the cholesterol/HDL-C and LDL-C/HDL-C ratios were significantly (p < 0.000, Tukey's HSD) higher in patients with major depression and patients in both phases of bipolar disorder than in healthy subjects. Moreover, patients with bipolar disorder in a depressive phase had a significantly (p = 0.045, Tukey's HSD) higher cholesterol/HDL-C ratio than bipolar patients in a manic phase and patients with major depression (p < 0.012, Tukey's HSD). In patients with bipolar disorder in a depressive phase the LDL-C/HDL-C ratio was also significantly (p = 0.01, Tukey's HSD) higher than in patients with major depression (Figure 2).

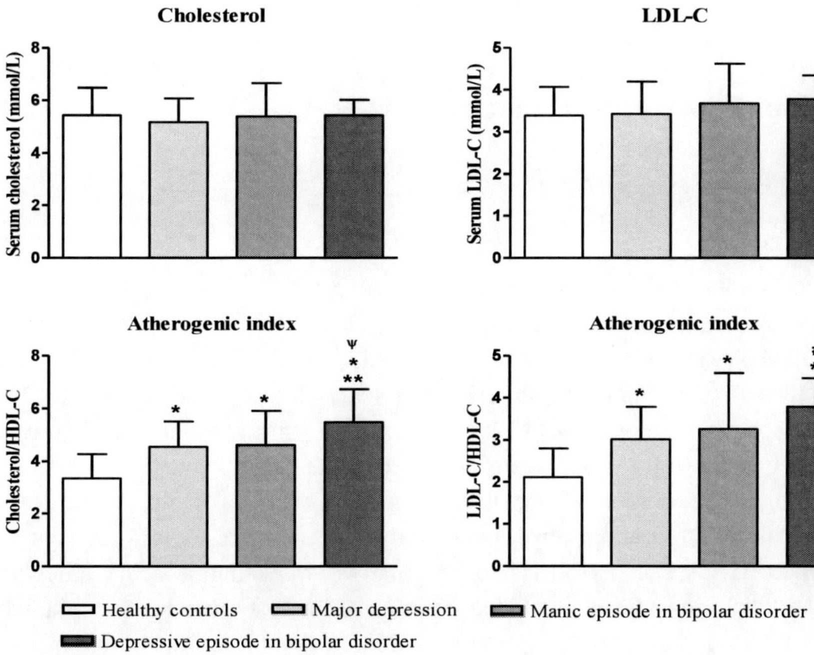

Figure 2. Serum cholesterol, LDL-C levels and atherogenic index (cholesterol/HDL-C and LDL-C/ HDL-C ratio) in healthy controls, patients with major depressive disorders, and patients with bipolar disorders in manic or depressive episodes. Results are expressed as means ± SD. *p < 0.000 vs. corresponding ratio in healthy controls; **p < 0.045 vs. cholesterol/HDL-C ratio in bipolar disorder in manic episode $^{\Psi}p$ < 0.012 vs. cholesterol/HDL-C ratio in major depression $^{\#}p$ <0.010 vs. LDL-C/HDL-C ratio in major depression (ANOVA followed by Tukey's test).

Table 4. Serum TG and HDL-C levels in healthy controls and in patients with major depressive or bipolar disorder

	Serum TG (mmol/L)	Serum HDL-C (mmol/L)
Healthy controls (50)	1.10 ± 0.37	1.66 ± 0.59
Patients with major depression (40)	1.35 ± 0.70	1.25 ± 0.36*
Patients with bipolar disorder		
- in manic episode (22)	1.70 ± 0.85*	1.22 ± 0.30*
- in depressive episode (19)	1.87 ± 0.85*,**	1.04 ± 0.28*

* $p < 0.05$ vs. corresponding values in healthy controls; **$p < 0.05$ vs. corresponding value in patients with major depression (Tukey's test).

3.2. Lipid Levels in Psychotic Mania

3.2.1. Subjects and Methods

Subjects

Forty male patients (age mean ± SD, 42.2 ± 14.1 years) with bipolar I disorder, current episode mania [Sagud et al., 2007], diagnosed according to the DSM-IV criteria [American Psychiatric Association, 1994], with more than 18 scores on Young Mania Rating Scale [YMRS; Young et al., 1978], and less than 7 scores on 17-item Hamilton Rating Scale for Depression [HAMD; Hamilton, 1960], were enrolled in the study. Patients with alcohol dependence, serious medical disease, recent change of the body weight, history of elevated cholesterol levels and on cholesterol-lowering drugs were excluded. Drug free period lasted at least two weeks. Benzodiazepines were allowed for nighttime sedation. Six patients had a first episode of mania, while two patients had a history of previous suicide attempt. Clinical characteristics of the patients are listed in Table 5.

The patients were further subdivided according to the score on item 8 (content) of YMRS into psychotic (score ≥ 5) and non-psychotic (score < 5) subgroups. Total YMRS scores were significantly ($p < 0.001$, Student's t-test) higher in psychotic (35.8 ± 7.6) than in non-psychotic (27.0 ± 4.6) manic patients. The number of recurrent episodes significantly correlated with age (r = 0.52; $p < 0.000$).

Table 5. The clinical characteristics of the patients with bipolar I disorder in manic phase

	mean ± SD
YMRS total scores	31.0 ± 7.1
HAMD total scores	1.7 ± 1.9
Duration of bipolar I disorder (years)	9.24 ± 8.85
Duration of current manic phase (days)	38.8 ± 40.6
Number of lifetime manic episodes	4.92 ± 5.83
Number of lifetime depressive episodes	4.73 ± 5.14

Age-matching control group (age mean ± SD, 36.8 ± 10.3 years) included 32 drug-free healthy men with no personal or familiar history of psychiatric disorders. Thirty patients and 8 healthy persons were smokers. Body mass index (BMI) was calculated by dividing weight (in kilograms) by squared height (in meters). Mean BMI was very similar ($t = 1.13$; $df = 70$; $p = 0.26$) between manic patients (25.3 ± 2.7 kg/m2) and healthy controls (25.6 ± 2.6 kg/m2). All subjects signed an informed consent and the study was approved by local Ethics Committee.

Methods

The determination of platelet serotonin concentration [Muck-Seler et al., 1996] and platelet monoamino-oxidase (MAO) activity [Krajl, 1965] was performed as previously described. Briefly, after an overnight fasting, blood (4 ml) was taken in a plastic syringe with 1 mL of ACD anticoagulant. The platelet serotonin concentration and MAO activity were measured spectrofluorimetrically. Platelet protein concentration was determined by the method of Lowry et al. (1951), while serum lipid levels were determined using standard laboratory methods.

Statistical Analysis

The results were expressed as mean ± SD. Student's t test, one-way analysis of variance (ANOVA) followed by Tukey's test, analysis of covariance (ANCOVA) and Pearson's coefficient of correlation were used for the statistical evaluation of the results. The statistical program used was SigmaStat 3.1.

Table 6. Platelet 5-HT concentration, serum cholesterol and LDL-C levels in healthy controls and in psychotic and non-psychotic patients with mania

	Platelet 5-HT (nmol/mg protein)	Serum cholesterol (mmol/L)	Serum LDL-C (mmol/L)
Healthy controls (32)	1.29 ± 0.31	5.7 ± 1.2	3.67 ± 0.8
Patients with mania (40)	1.42 ± 0.37	4.9 ± 1.0	2.94 ± 0.8
- psychotic (17)	1.51 ± 0.36*	4.8 ± 0.8*	2.79 ± 0.8 *
- non-psychotic (23)	1.30 ± 0.35	5.1 ± 1.2	3.11 ± 0.8

The results are expressed as mean ± S.D. with number of subjects in parentheses. *$p < 0.05$ vs. corresponding value in healthy controls and non-psychotic patients with mania (ANOVA and Tukey's test).

3.2.2. Results

As shown in Figure 3, serum cholesterol and LDL-C values were significantly lower in manic patients than in healthy controls, while no significant differences in HDL-C and TG levels were found. The platelet serotonin concentration (1.42 ± 0.37 nmol/mg protein) and platelet MAO activity (26.5 ± 17.0 nmol 4-HOQ/mg protein/h) in manic patients were not significantly different from serotonin concentration (1.29 ± 0.31 nmol/mg protein) and platelet MAO activity (21.2 ± 9.1 nmol 4-HOQ/mg protein/h) in control subjects. Moreover, there was no significant ($p > 0.05$) correlation between platelet serotonin concentration or platelet MAO activity and serum lipid levels in healthy controls or patients.

When patients were subdivided into psychotic and non-psychotic subgroups, serum cholesterol ($F = 4.56$; df = 2.69; $p = 0.014$) and LDL-C ($F = 8.21$; df = 2.69; $p = 0.001$), but not HDL-C and TG levels, significantly differed among groups. Namely, significantly lower ($p < 0.05$, Tukey's test) cholesterol and LDL values were observed in psychotic manic patients than in non-psychotic patients and healthy controls (Table 6). This significant difference persisted also when the data for cholesterol and LDL levels were adjusted for age ($F = 5.78$; $p = 0.001$, $F = 5.99$; $p = 0.001$,) and BMI ($F = 4.07$; $p = 0.01$, $F = 6.12$; $p = 0.001$) as covariates, respectively (ANCOVA). The results also demonstrated significant (p = 0.027, ANOVA) differences in platelet serotonin values, but not in the in platelet MAO activity, among psychotic and non-psychotic subgroups, with platelet serotonin concentration significantly higher ($p < 0.05$, Tukey's test) in psychotic patients then in non-psychotic patients and healthy subjects (Table 6). There was no significant ($p > 0.05$) correlation between platelet serotonin and cholesterol or LDL values in psychotic and non-psychotic patients, as well.

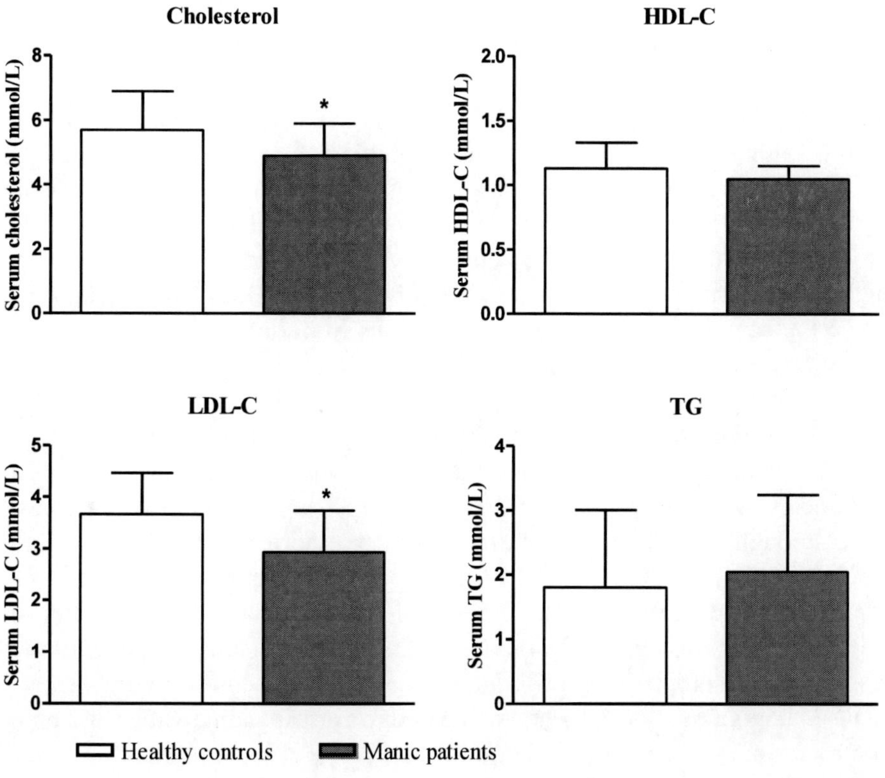

Figure 3. Serum cholesterol, high-density-lipoprotein cholesterol (HDL-C), low-density-lipoprotein cholesterol (LDL-C) and triglycerides (TG) levels in healthy controls (N = 32) and in manic patients (N= 40). Results are expressed as means ± SD. *$p < 0.01$ vs. corresponding values in the healthy controls (ANOVA following Tukey's test).

4. Lipids and Suicidal Behavior

A number of studies have shown a possible link between low levels of cholesterol and suicide [Lindberg et al., 1992; Neaton et al., 1992; Partonen et al., 1999; Lester, 2002; Muldoon et al., 1990; Fiedorowicz and Coryell, 2007; Zureik et al., 1996; Ellison and Morrison, 2001; Iribarren et al., 1995], with reduced cholesterol levels being associated with an increased risk of suicide [Partonen et al., 1999; Lindberg et al., 1992, Boston et al., 1996; Rabe-Jablonska and Poprawska, 2000; Sarchiapone et al., 2000]. Namely, serum cholesterol has been reported to be lower in subjects who attempted suicide compared to non-attempters in several studies [Golier et al., 1995; Kunugi et al., 1997; Papassotiropoulos et al., 1999; Garland et al., 2000, Modai et al., 1994], although some authors have failed to confirm these findings [Seneviratne et al., 1999; Almeida- Montes et al., 2000; Huang, 2005; Zhang et al., 2005]. The proportion of men who attempted suicide, or the proportion of patients with a first degree relative who completed suicide, was found higher in the subjects with lower cholesterol levels [Bocchetta et al., 2001], while the severity of a suicide attempt seems to be inversely correlated with serum cholesterol content [Kim et al., 2002]. Some studies also reported that the degree of suicidal ideation was inversely related to cholesterol levels [Papassotiropoulos et al., 1999; Sullivan et al., 1994]. There were also reports of low cholesterol levels among parasuicidal patients [Gallerani et al., 1995; Garland et al., 2000].

Although some authors reported a negative correlation between HDL-C levels and suicide attempts [Maes et al., 1997; Zhang et al., 2005], most studies point to LDL-C as the cholesterol fraction related to suicidality and self-harm. For instance, Agargun et al. (2004) found that patients with dissociative disorders and self-injurious behavior had lower serum levels of LDL-C, but not of HDL-C, when compared to corresponding values in healthy controls. Some other authors reported that, compared with controls, patients with self-harm had significantly lower levels of TC, LDL-C, and omega-3 fatty acids [Garland et al., 2007]. Several more studies demonstrated significantly lower TC and LDL-C levels in the suicidal group (Lee and Kim, 2003). On the other hand, studies in Korean populations have reported that serum TG levels tend to be lower among suicide attempters than non-suicidal patients with major depressive disorder [Kim et al., 2002; Lee and Kim, 2003; Kim and Myint, 2004].

In addition to suicide attempts and self-injurious [Kunugi et al., 1997; Alvarez et al., 1999; Garland et al., 2000; Diaz-Sastre et al., 2007;

Fiedorowicz and Coryell, 2007; Perez-Rodriguez et al., 2008; Atmaca et al., 2002b], serum total cholesterol has been also linked to violent behavior and impulsivity [Virkkunen, 1983; Golomb et al., 2000; Vevera et al., 2003] and violent method of suicide attempt [Alvarez et al., 2000; Atmaca et al., 2008; Fiedorowicz and Coryell, 2007]. Moreover, reduced levels of cholesterol in the brain have been found in violent suicide victims in a postmortem studies [Lalovic et al., 2007a,b]. The significant associations of hypocholesterolemia with violent and suicidal behavior were also found in subjects with disorders of lipoprotein metabolism, characterized by low cholesterol levels [Lalovic et al., 2004; Edgar et al., 2007]. Some studies demonstrated an increase in violence-related deaths, such as suicides, accidents, and homicides among individuals taking serum cholesterol-lowering medications [Frick et al., 1987; Muldoon et al., 1990], or among patients receiving trials of dietary interventions and non-statin drugs [Muldoon et al., 2001]. However, more recent studies did not reveal an association between lipid lowering medications and suicide [Lester, 2002; Callréus et al., 2007].

Other studies also suggested the relationship between low cholesterol levels, or lowering cholesterol by diet or medication, and aggression, violence and severe irritability [Golomb, 1998; Hillbrand et al., 2000]. Richards et al. (2000) found that disposition to experience and express anger was positively correlated with serum levels of TC and LDL-C. On the other hand, the study of Troisi and D'Argenio (2006) demonstrated that in control subjects with a low propensity toward aggressive behavior, higher levels of physical aggression and anger were correlated with lower levels of LDL-C. Among subjects who had recently committed a violent offence, physical aggression were positively correlated with LDL-C levels, while verbal aggression, anger and hostility were negatively correlated with HDL-C levels [Troisi and D'Argenio; 2006]. Positive correlations between pro-atherogenic cholesterol fractions and premeditated, but not impulsive aggression have been also observed [Conklin and Stanford, 2008]. Moreover, the increased propensity to engage in physical violence has been associated with lower concentrations of pro-atherogenic lipid and lipoprotein fractions [Chakrabarti and Sinha; 2006]. In addition, an increase in aggressive behavior has been observed in non-human primates assigned to low-cholesterol diets [Fontenot et al., 1996; Kaplan et al., 1991, 1994].

It has been indicated that the relation between aggression (directed toward either self or others) and cholesterol levels is largely attributable to a deficit in impulse control. Some studies demonstrated that subjects with low serum cholesterol show greater impulsivity [Pozzi et al., 2003]. Buydens-Branchey et al. (2000) found negative correlation between HDL-C levels and Barratt Impulsivity Scale (BIS). On the other hand, the results of some studies suggested that low concentrations of TC and LDL-C (but not HDL-C) were associated with increased impulsivity [Conklin and Stanford; 2008]. Garland et al. (2007) found that neither TC nor LDL-C alterations, but low levels of omega-3 and omega-6 fatty acids were associated with greater impulsivity scores. The modest increase in impulsivity was observed after a short course of cholesterol-lowering therapy that dissipated over a longer course of therapy [Ormiston et al., 2003].

4.1. Lipid Levels and Suicidal Behavior in Borderline Personality Disorder

4.1.1. Subjects and Methods

Subjects

Subjects included in the study were male patients, admitted to the Department of Psychiatry, University Hospital Zagreb, during the period of 12 months. The trained psychiatrists performed clinical evaluation [Marcinko et al., 2011]. The diagnosis of borderline personality disorder (BPD) was made according to diagnostic criteria of the International Statistical Classification of Diseases and Related Health Problems after structured diagnostic psychiatric interview for ICD-10 [WHO, 1992]. Within patients diagnosed with BPD, 20 of them were consecutively admitted men with suicidal behavior, while 20 patients were consecutively admitted men without suicidal behavior. The Brief Psychiatric Rating Scale [BPRS; Overall and Gorham, 1962] was used to assess a broad range of psychopathology. Patients were classified as suicidal if a suicidal ideation, or a suicide attempt, or both were present. Suicidality was defined if patients had 2 or more scores on the BPRS, on the item on suicide (item 4), while non-suicidal patients had score 1. Hamilton Depression Rating Scale, HDRS-17 [Hamilton, 1960] was used in order to assess depressive symptoms. Structured individual psychoanalytic psychotherapy prior to the hospitalization (during the previous 6 months) was detected in every patient, as well as the family history of suicidal behavior. All patients were free of all medications in the previous 3 weeks.

The control group included 20 healthy randomly selected male subjects with no history of psychiatric illness and suicidal behavior. None of the patients or control subjects included in the study had used any cholesterol-lowering drugs before the sampling. The exclusion criteria were: hypertension, hypothyroidism, diabetes mellitus, disorders of the lipoprotein metabolism, including alcoholism and eating disorders. All subjects were closely matched for age. The study was approved by the Medical Ethics Committee of Clinical Hospital Center and all participants gave their written informed consent to participate in the study.

Methods

Blood samples were collected from all subjects at 8.00 a.m. after an overnight fasting. Serum cholesterol concentration was determined enzymatically, using commercial kits (Olympus Diagnostic GmbH, Hamburg, Germany) on Olympus AU 600 automatic analyzer. Body mass index (BMI) was used as a marker of the dietary habits.

Statistical Analysis

The results were expressed as mean ± SD. Statistical analyses were performed with the SPSS statistical program, version 10 for Windows. The results were evaluated using one-way analysis of variance (ANOVA) followed by a Scheffee's multiple comparison test, or when two groups were compared using Student's t-test. Age and BMI were included as covariates within analysis of covariance (ANCOVA) in the comparison of serum cholesterol levels. The differences in the socio-demographic variables between suicidal and non-suicidal groups were assessed using a Chi square ($\chi 2$) test. *P*-values of < 0.05 were considered significant.

4.1.2. Results

No significant differences in the occurrence of the socio-demographic variables including those in the family and marital status, degree of education, employment and family history of suicidal behavior between suicidal and non-suicidal BPD patients were detected (data not shown). However, although these differences were not significant, suicidal patients, compared to non-suicidal patients, reported more cases of family history of suicidal behavior.

Age did not differ significantly ($p > 0.05$) between suicidal (mean ± SD, 29.00 ± 6.54 years) and non-suicidal patients (mean ± SD, 29.85 ± 7.57 years) and healthy subjects (mean ± SD, 32.10 ± 7.23 years). Moreover, there were no significant differences (ANOVA and Scheffe's test) in BMI, as well as in serum cholesterol levels, between suicidal and non-suicidal patients and healthy controls (Figure 4). These results remained the same after controlling for age and BMI (ANCOVA).

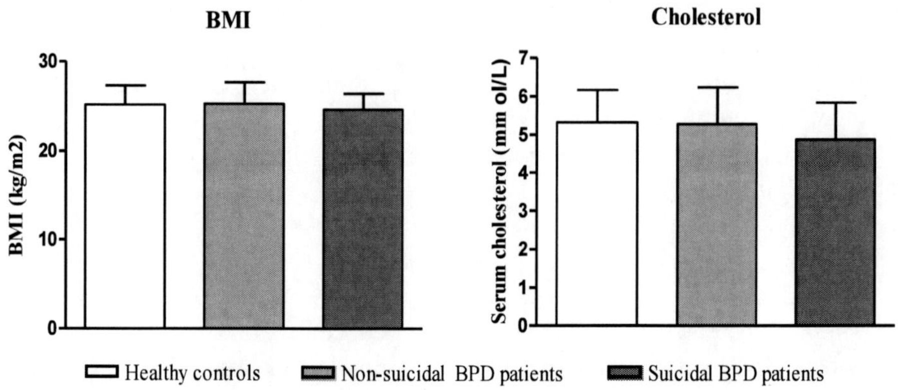

Figure 4. BMI and serum cholesterol levels (mean ± SD) in male suicidal (N = 20) and non-suicidal patients (N =20) with borderline personality disorder and in healthy control subjects (N = 20). Results are expressed as means ± SD.

As shown in Figure 5, HDRS-17 and BPRS scores were significantly (Student's t-test) higher in suicidal compared to non-suicidal patients. Seven out of 24 symptoms (anxiety, depression, suicidality, grandiosity, tension, excitement and motor hyperactivity) on BPRS were significantly higher in suicidal patients, compared to non-suicidal patients (Figure 5). There was no significant correlation between cholesterol and each symptom of the BPRS.

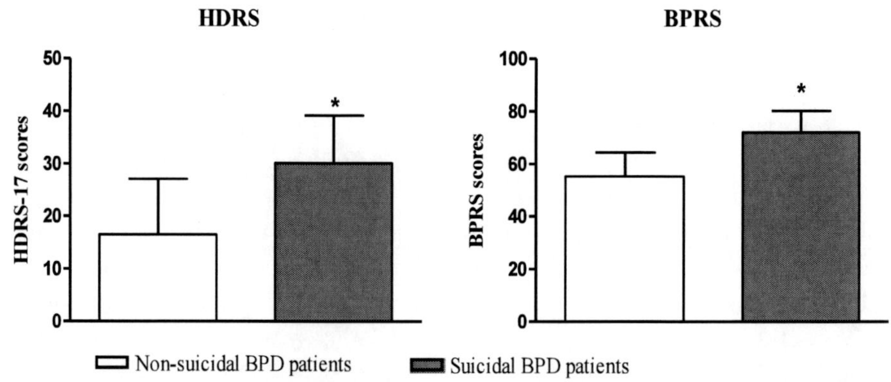

Figure 5. HDRS-17 and BPRS (mean ± SD) in male suicidal (N = 20) and non-suicidal patients (N = 20) with borderline personality disorder. Results are expressed as means ± SD.*p = 0.000 vs. non-**suicidal BPD patients** (Student's t-test).

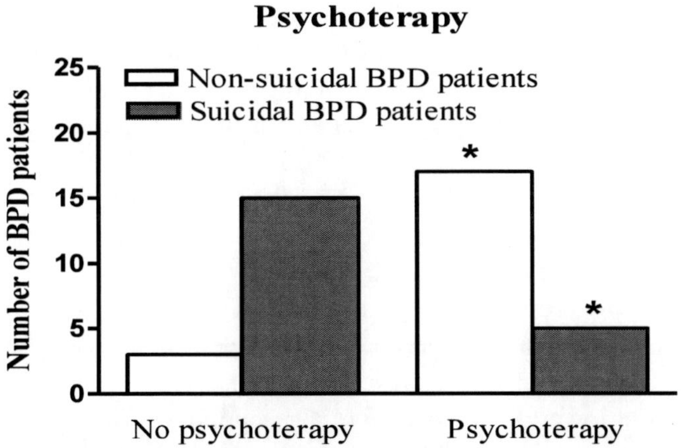

Figure 6. Structured individual psychoanalytic psychotherapy prior to the hospitalization for male suicidal (N = 20) and non-suicidal (N = 20) patients with borderline personality disorder. * $p = 0.000$ vs. group with no psychotherapy ($\chi 2$ test).

On the other hand, a significant ($\chi 2 = 14.545$; df = 1; $p = 0.000$) difference in the frequency of the structured individual psychoanalytic psychotherapy, received prior to the hospitalization, between suicidal and non-suicidal patients with BPD was observed. Namely, non-suicidal male patients with BPD received more frequently structured individual psychoanalytic psychotherapy prior to the hospitalization than suicidal group (Figure 6).

4.2. Lipid Levels and Suicidal Behavior in Psychotic Disorder

4.2.1. Subjects and Methods

Subjects

The study enrolled 54 male patients admitted to the Department of Psychiatry, Clinical Hospital Center Zagreb, during a period of 12 months [Marcinko et al., 2007]. The diagnosis of Psychotic Disorder Not Otherwise Specified (the first episode of psychosis) was made according to DSM-IV criteria, after performing the Structured Clinical Interview for DSM-IV [First et al., 1995]. Namely, the specified psychotic symptoms had been present for less than 1 month but had not yet remitted, so that the criteria for brief psychotic disorder were not met. The Hamilton Depression Rating Scale (HDRS-17) [Hamilton, 1960] was used for quantification of depressive symptoms. Within patients, 27 of them were consecutively admitted suicidal men in the first episode of psychosis (without suicidal anamnesis prior to psychotic episode), while 27 patients were consecutively admitted men in the first episode of psychosis, without suicidal behavior. Suicidality was positively defined if patients had 2 or more scores on the Brief Psychiatric Rating Scale (BPRS) on item on suicide (item 4). The BPRS [Overall and Gorham, 1962] was used to assess a broad range of psychopathology. All patients were free of all medications for previous 3 months.

For a control group 27 healthy male subjects with no history of psychiatric illness and suicidal behavior were randomly selected. The subjects in groups were closely matched by age. None of the patients or control subjects had used any cholesterol-lowering drugs before the sampling. The exclusion criteria were hypertension, hypothyroidism, diabetes mellitus, lipoprotein metabolism disorders, diagnosis of substance abuse including alcoholism, eating disorders and organic brain syndrome. The study was approved by the Clinical Hospital Center Medical Ethics Committee, and all subjects gave their written informed consent to participate in the study.

Methods

Blood samples were collected from all subjects at 8.00 a.m. after an overnight fasting. Immediately after the blood collection, the serum concentration of cholesterol was determined enzymatically by using commercial kits (Olympus Diagnostic GmbH, Hamburg, Germany) on an Olympus AU 600 automatic analyzer. The body mass index (BMI) was used as a marker of dietary habits. Platelet serotonin concentration was determined by the spectrofluorimetric method as previously described [Pivac et al., 1997]. The method of Lowry et al. (1951) was used for determination of total platelet protein concentrations.

Statistical Analysis

The results were expressed as mean ± S.D. One-way analysis of variance (ANOVA) followed by the Scheffé's multiple comparison test was used for the statistical evaluation of the results. Age and BMI were included as covariates within analysis of covariance (ANCOVA) in the comparison of serum cholesterol levels. P-values of < 0.05 were considered significant.

4.2.2. Results

No significant differences in age were observed between 27 suicidal patients (mean ± SD, 29.70 ± 7.22 years), 27 non-suicidal patients (mean ±

SD, 29.56 ± 8.67 years) and 27 healthy subjects (mean ± SD, 30.33 ± 3.13 years). The BMI (kg/m2) was very similar between suicidal, non-suicidal patients and control subjects, 25.77 ± 2.63, 26.24 ± 1.93 and 26.91 ± 2.09, respectively. Within patients in the fist episode of psychosis, the BPRS scores did not differ significantly (Student's t-test) between suicidal and non-suicidal patients (Figure 7). However, as shown in Figure 7, the HDRS-17 scores were significantly (Student's t-test) higher in suicidal compared to non-suicidal male patients.

Platelet serotonin concentration was significantly ($p = 0.000$ and $p = 0.002$, Scheffé's test, respectively) lower in suicidal than in non-suicidal patients, or in healthy controls (Figure 8). In addition, serum cholesterol levels were also significantly reduced ($p = 0.042$ and $p = 0.01$, Scheffé's test, respectively) in suicidal when compared to non-suicidal patients or healthy subjects (Figure 8). These differences remained after controlling for age and BMI ($p = 0.028$, ANCOVA).

No significant correlation was found between platelet serotonin concentration and cholesterol, or between platelet serotonin concentration and age in non-suicidal or suicidal patients or in healthy subjects. In addition, no significant correlation was detected between platelet serotonin levels and HDRS-17 scores, or platelet serotonin values and BPRS scores in non-suicidal or suicidal patients.

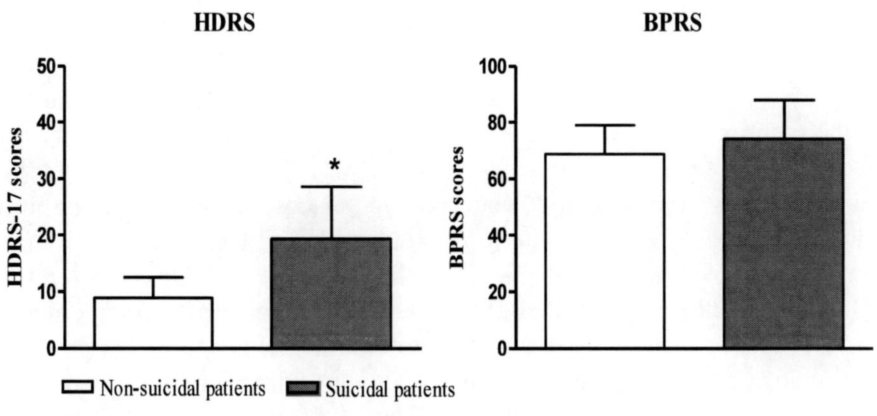

Figure 7. HDRS-17 and BPRS (mean ± SD) in male suicidal (N = 27) and non-suicidal patients (N = 27) with a first episode of psychosis. Results are expressed as means ± SD.*$p = 0.000$ vs. non-suicidal patients (Student's t-test).

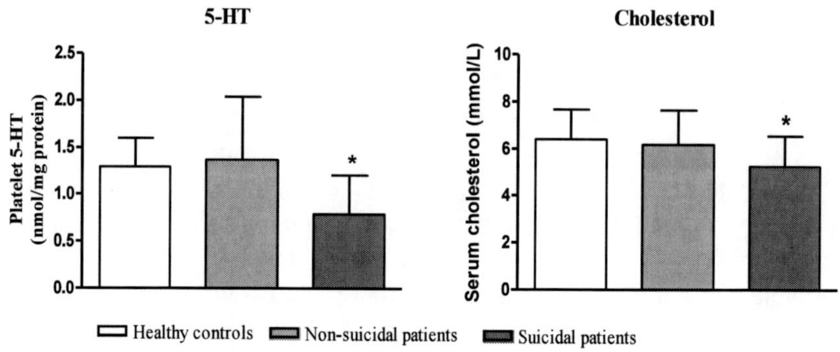

Figure 8. Platelet serotonin (5-HT) and serum cholesterol levels (mean ± SD) in male suicidal (N = 27) and non-suicidal (N = 27) patients with a first episode of psychosis and in healthy control subjects (N = 27). Results are expressed as means ± SD.$^*p <$ 0.05 vs. non-suicidal patients or healthy subjects (ANOVA followed by Scheffe's test).

5. Lipids and Serotonergic System

The relationship between lipid levels, neuropsychiatric disorders and treatment response is very complex. Most of the hypotheses trying to explain the association of cholesterol and mental health incorporate serotonin, proposing that elevated as well as low cholesterol levels may be associated with serotonergic dysfunction, which in turn is linked to a variety of neuropsychiatric disorders.

It has been proposed that low serum cholesterol may influence the fluidity of the neuronal cell membrane, consequently affecting the serotonergic neurotransmission [Engelberg, 1992]. Namely, reduced cholesterol in brain cell membranes would lead to lower lipid microviscosity, which could result in reduced number of pre-synaptic serotonin transporters or post-synaptic serotonin receptors being presented, resulting in decreased serotonin binding and uptake [Wallner and Machatschke, 2009; Engelberg, 1992]. An alternative model proposed that decrease in total cholesterol or LDL-C would induce a relative increase in brain cell membrane fluidity with increased presynaptic serotonin reuptake and decreased postsynaptic serotonin function [Diebold et al., 1998]. Kaplan et al. (1997) proposed an evolutionary rationale for the cholesterol–serotonin hypothesis suggesting that in conditions of decreased food intake and reduced cholesterol levels, lower serotonin levels would cause adaptive behavioral responses, including an increase in aggression and food competition.

A number of studies suggested that low cholesterol levels may affect mood and induce aggression, depression and suicidal behavior leading to completed suicide by modulating the serotonergic system [Fava, 1998; Fava and Rosenbaum, 1998; Fava et al., 2000, Hawton et al., 1993; Heron et al., 1980; Kaplan et al., 1997; Ringo et al., 1994; Golomb, 1998]. It has been hypothesized that a decrease in total serum cholesterol may lead to a decrease in brain serotonin levels [Steegmans et al., 1996]. In addition, a correlation between serum cholesterol and CSF 5-HIAA levels has been demonstrated in animal studies [Muldoon et al., 1992], although some studies in humans have not confirmed these findings [Ringo et al., 1994; Hibbeln et al., 2000].

Low cholesterol levels within cell membranes are associated with reduced binding affinity of a serotonin receptor agonist, altered G-protein coupling and decreased number of serotonin receptors, as well as reduced serotonin transporter activity [Engelberg, 1992; Scanlon et al., 2001 Papakostas et al 2004b; Pucadyil and Chattopadhyay, 2007]. Additionally, monkeys on a low-cholesterol diet had lower serotonin metabolite levels and lower central serotonergic activity than monkeys on a high-cholesterol diet [Muldoon et al., 1992; Kaplan et al., 1994]. A number of other studies have also suggested that serum cholesterol may be a limited marker for central serotonergic activity [Steegmans et al., 1996; Terao et al., 2000b; Vevera et al., 2005]. The lipid fraction associated with reduced serotonin function is HDL-C, while TC or LDL-C levels are not related to the serotonergic system [Buydens-Branchey et al., 2000]. On the other hand, Hibbeln et al. (1998) found a strong correlation between brain serotonin metabolites and omega-3 fatty acids, suggesting that cholesterol was acting as a ''surrogate marker'' for omega-3 fatty acids [Hibbeln et al., 2000].

Fischer et al. (2006) demonstrated the association of the short allele of the serotonin transporter polymorphism (5-HTTLPR) and LDL-C levels, with higher levels of LDL-C observed in individuals with the long allele than in individuals with the short allele. Moreover, many studies have shown that the short allele is a risk factor for a variety of psychiatric disorders [Serretti et al., 2006], while some studies reported greater risk for myocardial infarction in individuals with the long/long 5-HTTLPR genotype [Coto et al., 2003; Fumeron et al., 2002].

An alternative mechanism for the explanation of the relationship between depression and low cholesterol values was proposed [Maes et al., 1997]. Depressed patients with low HDL-C levels may actually have low activity of lecithin cholesterol acetyltransferase (LCAT), the enzyme responsible for the formation of most cholesterol esters in serum. Since the esterification of free cholesterol is important for the transport and elimination of free cholesterol from the body, patients with low LCAT activity, with low or even normal serum levels of cholesterol, could have decreased elimination of body cholesterol and an increase in the cholesterol content in the neuronal membrane, thereby adversely effecting neuronal structure and physiology [Maes et al., 1997].

Cholesterol-deficiency in neuronal membranes may also have a direct averse impact on dendritic outgrowth [Fan and Watanabe, 2000], synapse formation [Mauch et al., 2001], and even on neuronal survival [Michikawa and Yanagisawa, 1999]. Hence, another possible explanation is that decreased cholesterol in peripheral blood may result in reduced cholesterol levels in the brain, which may lead to reduced synaptic plasticity and brain dysfunction associated with neurobehavioral consequences [Mauch et al., 2001; Pfrieger, 2003].

Interleukin-2 (IL-2) has been also shown to cause a decrease in serum cholesterol while suppressing melatonin secretion from the pineal gland that, in turn, has been hypothesized to lead to depression and suicidal ideation [Penttinen, 1995].

Besides low cholesterol levels, elevated cholesterol levels may be also associated with serotonergic dysfunction [Fava et al., 2000]. Elevated cholesterol levels may lead to lower serotonin receptor sensitivity or serotonin transporter activity in depressed patients, either directly by binding to the various membrane-bound serotonin receptors or transporters, or indirectly by altering the fluidity of the neuronal membrane and thereby the conformation of these structures.

Some studies used meta-chlorophenylpiperazine (m-CPP) and D,L-fenfluramine as probes for serotonergic function [Kahn and Wetzler, 1991; Terao et al., 2000b; Meltzer and Maes, 1995; Coccaro et al., 1996]. Serum cholesterol levels are shown to be positively correlated with the degree of cortisol and prolactin secretion induced by administration of m-CPP and D,L-fenfluramine [Cowen, 1993], suggesting that a greater degree of sensitivity of serotonin receptors is associated with higher cholesterol levels and vice versa [Terao et al., 1997, 2000b]. Depressed patients with elevated cholesterol levels were more likely to demonstrate an attenuated cortisol and blunted prolactin response to m-CPP and D,L-fenfluramine [Papakostas et al., 2003a; 2004]. These findings are in accordance with reports that suggest the degree of serotonin receptor sensitivity, as evidenced by an elevated secretion of cortisol or prolactin after administration of D,L-fenfluramine or m-CPP, to confer a good prognosis to treatment [Malone et al., 1993; Cleare et al., 1998]. In line with these results, high cholesterol levels has been demonstrated in depressed patients with anger attacks [Fava et al., 1996], a population that also shows attenuated serotonergic function i.e. blunted prolactin response to D,L-fenfluramine [Fava et al., 2000].

It has been demonstrated that depressed patients with higher cholesterol levels were more likely to be non-responders to treatment with antidepressant drug fluoxetine, than patients with non-elevated cholesterol levels [Sonawalla et al., 2002]. Moreover, the patients with treatment resistant depression (TRD) had higher TG levels and a trend towards higher cholesterol levels, while high cholesterol levels predict poor response to nortriptyline in patients with TRD [Papakostas et al., 2003b]. As already mentioned, by interaction with serotonergic system, lipids modulate functional activity of the serotonin transporter [Allen et al., 2007], which is a target for numerous antidepressant drugs. Treatment with antidepressants and serotonin reuptake inhibitors (SSRI) have been associated with elevated cholesterol levels [Herran et al., 2006, Raeder et al., 2006; Meyer and Koro, 2004; Gabriel, 2007].

Elevated cholesterol levels are markers of vascular disease, which may be also associated with poor response to antidepressants. Several reports suggested that vascular risk factors (smoking, hypertension, and increased serum cholesterol) play an important role in the etiology of depression, and there is some neuropathological evidence demonstrating vascular changes in late life depression [Thomas et al., 2001]. Some studies suggest that high cholesterol levels result in blunted serotonin-mediated coronary arterial vasodilation [Cohen et al., 1988; Shimokawa and Vanhoutte, 1989; Lamping et al., 1999]. Patients with high cholesterol levels, due to familial combined hyperlipidemia (FCH), showed low platelet serotonin concentrations and low collagen-mediated serotonin release in their platelets, as well as blunted serotonin mediated vasodilation in forearm arteries, which normalized with lipid-lowering therapy [Stroes et al., 1995, 1997; Smith and Betteridge, 1997; O'Driscoll et al., 1997; Perticone et al., 2000].

Another possible explanation for the relationship between elevated cholesterol levels in depressed patients and treatment non-response may be that an excess of cholesterol in cell membranes enhances the activity of the enzyme γ-secretase in CNS neurons. In that way cholesterol inhibits neuronal and dendritic outgrowth and promotes the formation of beta-amyloid, implicated in the pathophysiology of Alzheimer's disease [Wahrle et al., 2002; Refolo et al., 2001; Shie et al., 2002].

5.1. Lipid Levels and Treatment Response to Antidepressants

5.1.1. Subjects and Methods

Subjects

Sixty non-suicidal, non-psychotic, female inpatients (age mean ± SD, 52.6 ± 10.8 years; range 36 - 59 years) with major depression diagnosed using a semistructured clinical interview according to the DSM-IV criteria [American Psychiatric Association, 1994], were included in the study [Muck-Seler et al., 2011]. Exclusion criteria were change (± 5%) in body weight in the previous 3 months; use of cholesterol-lowering drugs; hyperlipidemia, pregnancy; lactation; suicidal ideation; alcohol/drug abuse in previous month; other axis I psychiatric disorders; serious medical conditions; additional psychotropic drugs, electroconvulsive therapy or intensive psychotherapy, and clinical symptoms of hyperthyroidism or hypothyroidism. All patients were medication free for at least 14 days, and 18 patients received no pharmacological treatment for more than 8 weeks. Benzodiazepines were allowed if necessary.

In an open, randomized study, 33 and 27 patients were treated with paroxetine (20 mg/day) and tianeptine (3 x 12.5 mg/day), respectively. Fifteen patients treated with paroxetine and eleven treated with tianeptine were in menopause. At baseline, patients treated with paroxetine or tianeptine were matched ($p > 0.05$, ANOVA) on duration of illness, number of previous episodes and duration of the present episode (Table 7). As shown in Table 7, they did not differ significantly ($p > 0.05$) in age, body mass index and HDRS scores.

Moreover, baseline serum lipid levels were similar ($p > 0.05$) in patients treated with paroxetine or tianeptine, including total cholesterol (5.59 ± 0.84 or 5.80 ± 0.96 mmol/L), HDL-C (1.29 ± 0.37 or 1.27 ± 0.34 mmol/L), LDL- C (3.35 ± 1.17 or 3.86 ± 0.94 mmol/L), and TG (1.64 ± 0.64 or 1.87 ± 0.89 mmol/L).

The severity of depression was evaluated with 17-item Hamilton Depression Rating Scale (HDRS) [Hamilton, 1960] before and after 4 weeks of treatment with paroxetine or tianeptine. Responders to treatment were patients who had at least a 50 % reduction in the initial HDRS scores.

Table 7. The demographic and clinical characteristics of the patients with major depression before treatment with paroxetine or tianeptine

	Paroxetine group (N= 33)	Tianeptine group (N=27)
Age/Mean ± SD (range)	55.6 ± 9.5	50.3 ± 12.0
Body mass index (BMI) (kg/m^2)	25.2 ± 3.8	25 ± 2.7
Duration of illness (years)	6.2 ± 7.5	5.7 ± 6.6
Number of previous episodes	3.1 ± 3.3	3.2 ± 2.2
Duration of the present episode (months)	3.1 ± 1.9	2.5 ± 1.1
HDRS scores	27.0 ± 2.4	26.6 ± 2.0

All participants signed the written informed consent, while the study was performed in accordance with the Helsinki Declaration and approved by the local ethics committee.

Methods

Blood samples of the patients were drawn in the morning after an overnight fasting for 12 hours. For determination of serum cholesterol, HDL-C and TG levels the enzymatic color test for clinical analyzers was used, with the linearity within concentrations range of 0.64 to 18 mmol/L, 0.05 to 4.65 mmol/L and 0.11 to 11.40 mmol/L for serum cholesterol, HDL-C, and TG, respectively. Serum LDL-C levels were determined by using enzymatic clearance assay, with linearity up to 22.4 mol/L.

Statistical Analysis

The results are expressed as mean ± SD. Statistical analyses were performed with SigmaStat 3.1 The statistical evaluation of the data included one-way analysis of variance (ANOVA), Tukey post hoc test, analysis of covariance with age and menstrual status as covariates, and χ^2 test. The results were considered significant when $p < 0.05$.

5.1.2. Results

Following 4 weeks of treatment, good therapeutic response was observed in 22 (67%) of 33 paroxetine-treated patients and in 12 (44%) of 27 tianeptine-treated patients. The frequency of responders and nonresponders was similar ($\chi^2 = 2.15$; $p = 0.143$) between both treatment groups.

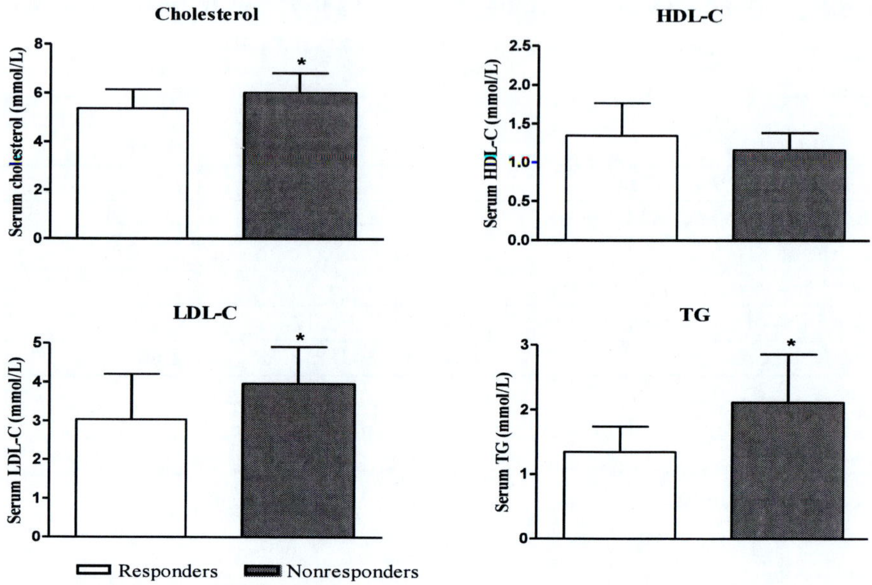

Figure 9. Pretreatment serum lipid levels in female patients with depression subdivided into responders (N = 22) and nonresponders (N = 11) to paroxetine treatment. The results are expressed as mean ± SD. The number of subjects is given in parentheses. $^{*}p < 0.05$ versus matching responders.

As expected, the total mean HDRS scores differed significantly in responders and nonresponders to both paroxetine and tianeptine treatment. Namely, the HDRS cores in nonresponders (22.0 ± 5.0) were significantly ($p <$ 0.05) higher then in responders (7.1 ± 4.7) to paroxetine treatment. Similarly, the HDRS cores in responders (5.5 ± 3.7) and nonresponders (25.6 ± 4.8) to tianeptine treatment were also significantly different.

Pretreatment serum cholesterol, TG, and LDL-C levels were significantly higher in nonresponders compared with responders to paroxetine treatment (Figure 9), and they were higher than normal values [Sagud et al., 2007]. The significant difference in total cholesterol ($p = 0.033$), TG ($p = 0.003$), and LDL-C ($p = 0.034$) levels persisted also when data were adjusted for age and menstrual status as covariates. On the other hand, there were no significant differences in the baseline serum HDL-C levels between responders and nonresponders to paroxetine treatment (Figure 9).

As shown in Figure 10, baseline lipid levels did not differ significantly ($p > 0.05$) between responders and nonresponders to tianeptine treatment.

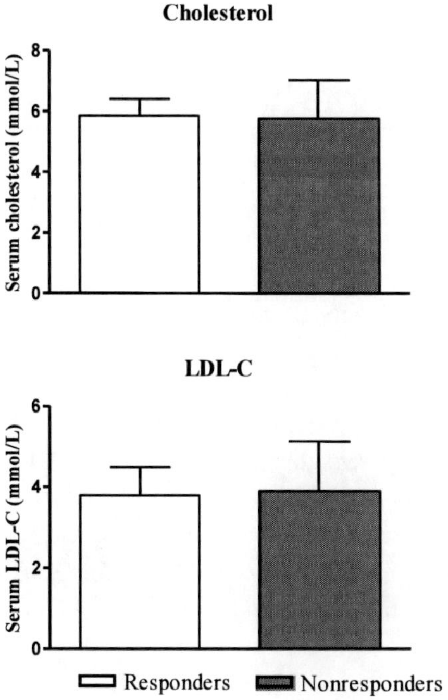

Figure 10. Pretreatment serum lipid levels in female patients with depression subdivided into responders (N = 12) and nonresponders (N = 15) to tianeptine treatment. The results are expressed as mean ± SD. The number of subjects is given in parentheses.

5.2. Lipid Levels and Serotonin Receptor Gene Polymorphisms

5.2.1. Subjects and Methods

Subjects

A total of 348 unrelated Caucasian subjects of Croatian origin, including 188 female and 160 male subjects were enrolled in the study. All subjects completed questionnaires regarding their medical history and smoking habits. All participants agreed to give a blood sample, to participate in the study, and gave their written informed consent. The study was approved by the local Ethics committee of the Institute for Medical Research and Occupational Health and was carried out in accordance with the Helsinki declaration of 1975.

Methods

Blood samples of the patients were drawn in the morning after an overnight fasting for 12 hours in plastic syringes with (for the isolation of DNA) or without EDTA coagulant (for determination of serum cholesterol, HDL-C and TG levels). Genomic DNA was isolated from peripheral blood leukocytes according to standard procedures by a salting out method. 5-HT1B, 5-HT2A and 5-HT2C receptor gene polymorphisms (rs13212041, rs6313 and rs3813929) were genotyped using Taqman^{TM} probe-primer combinations available from the Applied Biosystems Assay-on-Demand^{TM} human SNP genotyping collection (Applied Biosystems, Foster City, CA, USA). Taqman-based allele-specific polymerase chain reactions and post-PCR fluorescence plate reads were performed according to the procedure described by Applied Biosystems, using an ABI Prism 7000 Sequencing Detection System apparatus. Briefly, 20 ng of genomic DNA was PCR amplified in 96-well plates using a 5 μl reaction volume for 40 cycles at 92°C for 15 s followed by 60°C for 60 s. Serum lipid levels were determined enzymatically on COBAS Mira automatic analyzer by using standard laboratory methods.

Statistical Analysis

The results were expressed as mean ± SD. Statistical analyses were performed with the SigmaStat 2.0 (Jandel Scientific Corp., San Raphael, California, USA) and SPSS v. 13.01, statistical programs. The results were evaluated using one-way analysis of variance (ANOVA) followed by Newman-Keuls test or Student's t-test. *P*-values of < 0.05 were considered significant.

5.2.2. Results

The results demonstrated significantly higher levels of total serum cholesterol ($p < 0.001$), HDL-C ($p = 0.004$) and TG ($p = 0.012$), but significantly lower levels of LDL-C ($p = 0.001$) in female subjects, when compared to male subjects (Table 8).

When the serum lipid levels in subjects of both gender carrying AA, AG or GG genotypes of the 1997 A/G polymorphism in the 5-HT1B receptor gene were investigated, male carriers of AG genotype had significantly ($p < 0.05$) higher levels of cholesterol when compared with the cholesterol levels in AA genotype carriers (Table 9).

Table 8. Serum cholesterol, HDL-C, LDL-C and TG levels in female and male subjects

Serum Lipid levels	All subjects (348)	Female subjects (188)	Male subjects (160)
Cholesterol (mmol/L)	5.39 ± 1.67	5.68 ± 1.19 **	5.06 ± 1.05
HDL-C (mmol/L)	1.22 ± 0.40	1.29 ± 0.39**	1.14 ± 0.39
LDL-C (mmol/L)	3.40 ± 1.08)	3.06 ± 1.02 **	3.16 ± 1.09
TG (mmol/L)	1.61 ± 0.72	1.70 ± 0.74 *	1.50 ± 0.70

The results are expressed as mean ± S.D. with number of subjects in parentheses. *$p <$ 0.05, **$p < 0.005$ vs. corresponding value in male subjects (Student's t-test)

Table 9. Serum cholesterol, HDL-C, LDL-C and TG levels in female and male subjects carrying different genotypes of 5-HT1B receptor gene polymorphism

	5-HT1B receptor gene polymorphism genotype			*p*-value
	AA	AG	GG	
Serum cholesterol (mmol/L)	5.33 ± 1.21 (225)	5.53 ± 1.09 (115)	5.30 ± 1.03 (8)	0.315
Female subjects	5.72 ± 1.23 (119)	5.61 ± 1.14 (63)	5.64 ± 0.88 (6)	0.857
Male subjects	4.90 ± 1.02 (106)	5.43 ± 1.02 (52)*	4.28 ± 0.90 (2)	0.005
Serum HDL-C (mmol/L)	1.21 ± 0.38 (225)	1.25 ± 0.44 (115)	1.23 ± 0.24 (8)	0.682
Female subjects	1.31 ± 0.40 (119)	1.28 ± 0.39 (63)	1.25 ± 0.25 (6)	0.878
Male subjects	1.11 ± 0.32 (106)	1.22 ± 0.50 (52)	1.19 ± 0.28 (2)	0.245
Serum LDL-C (mmol/L)	3.40 ± 1.05 (223)	3.40 ± 1.14 (114)	3.41 ± 0.93 (8)	0.999
Female subjects	3.66 ± 1.06 (118)	3.50 ± 0.96 (63)	3,68 ± 0.79 (6)	0.580
Male subjects	3.11 ± 0.96 (105)	3.28 ± 1.33 (51)	2,60 ± 1.05 (2)	0.516
Serum TG (mmol/L)	1.57 ± 0.84 (225)	1.69 ± 1.44 (115)	1,44 ± 0.51(8)	0.247
Female subjects	1.71 ± 0.82 (119)	1.84 ± 0.87 (63)	1,57 ± 0.52 (6)	0.690
Male subjects	1.49 ± 0.84 (106)	1.89 ± 1.41 (52)	1,08 ± 0.28 (2)	0.242

The results are expressed as mean ± S.D. with number of subjects in parentheses. *$p <$ 0.05 vs. corresponding value in male subjects carrying AA genotype (ANOVA and Newman-Keuls test).

On the other hand, there were no significant differences in lipid levels between subjects of both sexes carrying CC, CT or TT genotypes of the 5-HT2A receptor gene polymorphism (Table 10).

As shown in the Table 11 and Table 12, there were no significant differences in serum lipid levels in male or in female subjects carrying different genotypes or alleles of 5-HT2C receptor gene polymorphism.

Table 10. Serum cholesterol, HDL-C, LDL-C and TG levels in female and male subjects carrying different genotypes of 5-HT2A receptor gene polymorphism

	5-HT2A receptor gene polymorphism genotype			*p*-value
	CC	CT	TT	
Serum cholesterol (mmol/L)	5.26 ± 1.15 (127)	5.49 ± 1.14 (163)	5.42 ± 1.28 (58)	0.252
Female subjects	5.58 ± 1.12 (65)	5.73 ± 1.21 (90)	5.73 ± 1.27 (33)	0.722
Male subjects	4.93 ± 1.08 (62)	5.19 ± 0.96 (73)	5.03 ± 1.20 (25)	0.340
Serum HDL-C (mmol/L)	1.21 ± 0.38 (127)	1.27 ± 0.43 (163)	1.14 ± 0.33 (58)	0.080
Female subjects	1.30 ± 0.39 (65)	1.34 ± 0.40 (90)	1.17 ± 0.36 (33)	0.104
Male subjects	1.10 ± 0.35 (62)	1.19 ± 0.44 (73)	1.10 ± 0.29 (25)	0.387
Serum LDL-C (mmol/L)	3.28 ± 1.10 (125)	3.47 ± 1.05 (162)	3.49 ± 1.07 (58)	0.271
Female subjects	3.54 ± 0.89 (64)	3.63 ± 1.10 (90)	3.67 ± 1.07 (33)	0.800
Male subjects	3.00 ± 1.04 (61)	3.26 ± 0.97 (72)	3.24 ± 1.03 (25)	0.361
Serum TG (mmol/L)	1.69 ± 1.06 (127)	1.66 ± 0.88 (163)	1.76 ± 0.88 (58)	0.757
Female subjects	1.73 ± 0.74 (65)	1.68 ± 0.83 (90)	1.96 ± 0.99 (33)	0.642
Male subjects	1.66 ± 1.33 (62)	1.62 ± 0.95 (73)	1.50 ± 0.62 (25)	0.877

The results are expressed as mean ± S.D. with number of subjects in parentheses.

Table 11. Serum cholesterol, HDL-C, LDL-C and TG levels in female subjects carrying different genotypes of 5-HT2C receptor gene polymorphism

	5-HT2C receptor gene polymorphism genotype			*p*- value
	CC	CT	TT	
Serum cholesterol (mmol/L)	5.71 ± 1.20 (125)	5.65 ± 1.20 (57)	5.31 ± 1.12 (6)	0.707
Serum HDL-C (mmol/L)	1.29 ± 0.39 (125)	1.32 ± 0.42 (57)	1.20 ± 0.21 (6)	0.739
Serum LDL-C (mmol/L)	3.61 ± 1.05 (125)	3.61 ± 0.95 (56)	3.44 ± 1.13 (6)	0.921
Serum TG (mmol/L)	1.78 ± 0.87 (125)	1.71 ± 0.77 (57)	1.46 ± 0.37 (6)	0.649

The results are expressed as mean ± S.D. with number of subjects in parentheses.

Table 12. Serum cholesterol, HDL-C, LDL-C and TG levels in male subjects carrying different alleles of 5-HT2C receptor gene polymorphism

	5-HT2C receptor gene polymorphism allele		*p*- value
	C	T	
Serum cholesterol (mmol/L)	5.10 ± 0.38(126)	4.93 ± 0.99 (34)	0.563
Serum HDL-C (mmol/L)	1.13 ± 0.39 (126)	1.21 ± 0.43 (34)	0.511
Serum LDL-C (mmol/L)	3.18 ± 1.13 (124)	3.07 ± 0.96 (34)	0.866
Serum TG (mmol/L)	1.67 ± 1.14 (126)	1.43 ± 0.76(34)	0.223

The results are expressed as mean ± S.D. with number of subjects in parentheses.

6. Discussion

Our results obtained on female patients with Alzheimer's disease demonstrated that serum lipid levels (total cholesterol, TG, HDL-C and LDL-C) are reduced in patients with Alzheimer's disease compared to elderly female healthy subjects, with the lowest serum lipid levels found in the late stage of Alzheimer's disease [present study, Presecki et al., 2011]. Namely, we have found significantly lower serum cholesterol and LDL-C levels in patients in the late phase of Alzheimer's disease compared to levels in patients in the middle phase of Alzheimer's disease. The alterations in serum lipid levels were independent on the presence of psychotic features.

Reduced serum cholesterol, LDL-C and HDL-C levels in patients with Alzheimer's disease have been observed also in some previous reports [Solfrizzi et al., 2006; Reitz et al., 2004; Merched et al., 2000]. However, in contrast to our results some authors reported elevated levels of LDL-C, increased or unaltered levels of cholesterol, as well as unaltered TG levels in patients with Alzheimer's disease [Kuo et al., 1998; Bonarek et al., 2000; Lesser et al., 2009; Mielke et al., 2005]. Our results demonstrating significantly lower TG levels in patients with Alzheimer's disease, especially in the late phase of the disease, suggest that TG could be involved in the progress of Alzheimer's disease. Moreover, to the best of our knowledge, these are the first reports of the significantly lower serum cholesterol and LDL-C levels in patients in the late phase of Alzheimer's disease compared to levels in patients in the middle phase of Alzheimer's disease.

On the other hand, there were no significant differences in lipid profile between patients with and without psychotic features, as well as no association between lipid levels and psychotic features, although it is known that psychotic features that distress patients, could be associated with the rapid progression of Alzheimer's disease [Schenider and Dagerman, 2004].

The contradictory data regarding lipid levels found in different studies might be due to the variety of factors including age, gender, diet, alcohol, exercise, smoking and different methods for the determination of lipid levels. For instance, different methods, such as enzymatic [Merched et al., 2000; present study] or high performance gel filtration chromatography [Kuo et al., 1998], were used for the determination of serum lipid levels. Besides, many studies have not specified the severity or the phases of the Alzheimer's disease in their patients [Kuo et al., 1998; Reitz et al., 2004; Merched et al., 2000]. In addition, a number of studies did not specify the gender of patients with Alzheimer's disease [Kuo et al., 1998] or have reported lipid levels in the groups of patients and controls that consisted of both male and female subjects [Reitz et al., 2004, Merched et al., 2000].

All these different factors made comparisons between studies even more difficult. Hence, in order to avoid the gender-related differences which have been observed not only in lipid levels (cholesterol, HDL-C, LDL-C and TG) in healthy subjects [Frikke-Schmidt et al., 2000; Wolf et al., 2004], but also in the clinical presentation [Grossi et al., 2005] and cognitive deficits [McPherson et al., 1999] in patients with Alzheimer's disease, our studies included only female subjects. The other advantages of the presented results were in ethnically uniform Caucasian sample of the control subjects as well as patients with Alzheimer's disease; and in carefully matched patients with elderly control group in terms of race, age, gender and in determination of all components of the lipid profile.

Although the patients in the late stage of Alzheimer's disease were the oldest, there were no significant correlations between age and lipid levels, suggesting no influence of aging on serum lipid levels. These results are in line with the findings of other studies on patients with Alzheimer's disease [Eckert et al., 2005], although aging has been associated with the decline in cholesterol synthesis in hippocampus of healthy subjects [Thelen et al., 2006].

In the present findings significant differences were detected in total lipid levels among patients with diverse degrees of the cognitive impairment. The results demonstrated that the difference in lipid levels among healthy controls and patients with Alzheimer's disease is due to the low serum lipid profile in patients with Alzheimer's disease in the late stage of the disease. Namely, all components of lipid profile were significantly lower in patients in the late stage of Alzheimer's disease then in healthy controls.

A significant decrease in cholesterol and LDL-C was also found in the late stage of Alzheimer's disease compared to lipid values in the middle phases of disease. Positive correlation between MMSE scores and cholesterol and LDL-C levels was observed in patients with Alzheimer's disease, suggesting the association of more severe symptoms of Alzheimer's disease with reduced cholesterol and LDL-C values. Although serum lipid levels were determined only in patients with Alzheimer's disease that were in middle or late stage of disease, the positive correlation between MMSE scores and serum cholesterol and LDL-C levels suggests that increased levels of those lipids could be the protective factor in the occurrence of Alzheimer's disease. These results are in line with the findings that increased plasma cholesterol levels are associated with a reduced risk of dementia in older subjects [Mielke et al., 2005], but are in contrast with the reports showing a positive [Notkola et al., 1998; Kivipelto et al., 2002] or non-significant [Tan et al., 2003; Li et al., 2005] association between high cholesterol and HDL-C levels in midlife and the development of Alzheimer's disease in the late life. The data on blood lipid levels and incidence of Alzheimer's disease seem to vary over the life course or in relation to the underlying course of Alzheimer's disease [Panza et al., 2006]. Low HDL-C levels have been associated with poor memory and progressive decline in memory in the middle aged adults [Singh-Manoux et al., 2008], while elevated HDL-C could be related to decreased incidence of dementia [Bonarek et al., 2000]. It is also possible that dementia itself modifies lipid levels, due to the changes in diet or metabolism, leading to low lipid levels in patients with Alzheimer's disease. Namely, it is known that diet could partially influence the serum lipid levels [Shobab et al., 2005]. However, in contrast to the uncontrolled dietary habits of the patients in middle stage of Alzheimer's disease, patients in the late stage of Alzheimer's disease, who had the lowest lipid levels, were hospitalized and fed with the balanced hospital diet. Therefore, for the patients in the late stage of Alzheimer's disease influence of the diet might be excluded.

Our results demonstrating reduced serum lipid levels in Alzheimer's disease are also in agreement with the reduced cholesterol and HDL-C levels in cerebrospinal fluid [Mulder et al., 1998], low hippocampal membrane cholesterol levels [Abad-Rodriguez et al., 2004], decreased activity of enzyme seladin-1, an enzyme involved in cholesterol synthesis [Ledesma et al., 2005], and reduced concentration of plasma 24S-hydroxycholesterol levels, a marker for the brain cholesterol metabolism [Solomon et al., 2009], observed in patients with Alzheimer disease. Although one might argue that peripheral cholesterol content does not contribute to the brain cholesterol levels, since plasma lipoproteins are unable to cross lipophilic blood-brain barrier [Shobab et al., 2005], and that there are many differences between cholesterol metabolism in the brain and periphery [Panza et al., 2006], a net flux of peripheral cholesterol in the form of 27-hydroxycholesterol through blood-brain-barrier was reported recently in healthy volunteers [Heverin et al., 2007], that could contribute to the cholesterol homeostasis in the brain through its effect on several cholesterol-sensitive genes.

Furthermore, the results of our other study suggested that lower HDL-C values and a higher atherogenic index (cholesterol/ HDL-C and LDL-C/HDL-C), observed in patients with major depression and bipolar disorder (both in a manic and a depressed episode) might represent a hallmark of affective disorders. These results are in line with the studies demonstrating association between low HDL-C levels and major depression [Maes et al., 1997; Huang, 2005], and also agree with the hypothesis that HDL-C might be a trait, rather than a state marker in bipolar disorders [Sobczak et al., 2004].

Our results also demonstrated higher TG levels in patients with bipolar disorder [Sagud et al., 2009], both in a manic and a depressed phase, compared with patients with major depression or healthy subjects. The slight increase in TG values also observed in patients with major depression is in agreement with the findings of Huang (2005), who reported higher TG levels in female patients with major depression. Plasma TG concentrations are suggested as important players in the content and distribution of HDL subclasses [Yang et al., 2005]. Although we have not determined the HDL subclasses in our study, our findings of increased TG and decreased HDL-C levels suggest a larger production of smaller-sized HDL particles [Yang et al., 2005], altered reverse cholesterol transport and abnormal HDL production in the patients with bipolar disorders.

Although a number of studies reported alterations in cholesterol and LDL-C levels in major depression and bipolar disorders [Maes et al., 1997; Ghaemi et al., 2000; Atmaca et al., 2002a; Cassidy and Carroll, 2002; Pae et al., 2004; Sagud et al., 2007], we found no significant changes between patients and control subjects, suggesting that both cholesterol and LDL-C levels are not related to diagnostic entities such as major depression or bipolar disorder. The discrepancies among studies might be due to various factors, including sex, medication status [Maes et al., 1997], decreased appetite/ weight loss [Boston et al., 1996], and suicide attempts [Marcinko et al., 2007].

As in the case of our study on patients with Alzheimer disease, the association between HDL-C levels and major depression and bipolar disorders was detected in only female subjects [present study, Sagud et al., 2019], avoiding possible influence of gender on lipid levels, which has been found in healthy subjects in several studies [Sudhop, 1999; Zhang et al., 2005]. Hence, lower HDL-C levels observed in our patients were not due to the sex-differences. Some studies suggested that lower HDL-C values might be also influenced by suicidal behavior in depressed man but not in depressed women [Maes et al., 1997]. However, as in our study the patients with a recent suicidal attempt were excluded, lower HDL-C levels could not be associated with a history of suicidal behavior.

The different data regarding lipid status might be also due to variations in medication status of patients, as numerous psychoactive drugs influence lipid levels [Weisler et al., 2005; Saari et al., 2004]. For instance, both treatment with antidepressants [Maes et al., 1997] and psychoactive drugs [Glueck et al., 1994] have been reported to significantly decrease serum cholesterol and HDL-C levels in patients with mood disorders. However, as subjects included in our study were medication-free females who did not show suicidal behavior, with no significant differences in BMI between groups; our results support the suggestion that cholesterol levels could not be a good biological marker for major depression [Oxenkrug et al., 1983].

Since HDL-C has a role in reverse cholesterol transport and complex cholesterol homeostasis, processes important in the protection of the cardiovascular system [Norata et al., 2006; Sampietro et al., 2006], our results demonstrating low HDL-C and high TG levels, might suggest that patients with mood disorders have a higher risk for the development of cardiovascular disorders [Lesperance et al., 1996; Polk and Naqui, 2005], such as coronary heart disease [Wilson et al., 1998; Franceschini, 2001], and should be followed up medically.

On the other hand, lower HDL-C levels might be also the result of altered serotonergic function [Buydens-Branchey et al., 2000]. Namely, different studies reported positive correlations between HDL-C levels and the serotonin metabolite 5-hydroxyindoleacetic acid in suicide attempters [Engstromet al., 1995], altered platelet serotonin in patients with bipolar disorder [Sagud et al., 2007], and inverse relationship between platelet serotonin and suicidal behavior in depressed patients [Muck-Seler et al., 1996; Pivac et al., 1997].

Hence, the next findings describe simultaneously compared platelet serotonin content, platelet MAO activity and serum lipid levels in drug free patients with bipolar disorder in a manic phase and psychotic and non-psychotic subtypes [present study, Sagud et al., 2007]. To eliminate the gender differences observed in lipid levels [Sudhop, 1999; Zhang et al., 2005], and platelet 5-HT values in healthy persons [Oxenkrug, 1979; Muck-Seler et al., 1996; Pivac et al., 2004] and psychiatric patients [Muck-Seler et al., 1996; Pivac et al., 2001; Pivac et al., 2004], our protocol included only male subjects.

Our results, demonstrating no significant differences in platelet serotonin concentration between manic patients and healthy controls, are in the contrast with studies showing increased [Saxena et al., 1999] or decreased [Takahashi, 1976] platelet serotonin concentrations in mania. However, both male and female patients were included in these studies [Takahashi, 1976; Saxena et al., 1999], while only male subjects participated in our study. Moreover, in contrast to a relatively small number of patients with mild or moderate symptoms of mania enrolled in the above-mentioned studies, our study included a considerable number of patients in a severe manic state.

In addition, our findings revealed different platelet serotonin concentrations between psychotic and non-psychotic subtypes of mania. These results are in line with studies reporting increased platelet serotonin concentration in other psychiatric disorders with psychotic features [Stahl et al., 1983; Muck-Seler et al, 1991; Muck-Seler et al., 1996; Meszaros et al., 1998; Pivac et al., 2006b]. Increased platelet serotonin concentration in psychotic mania might be the consequence of altered platelet serotonin uptake. However, inconsistent results showing decreased [Marazziti et al., 1991], increased [Meagher et al., 1990], or unchanged [Modai et al., 1984] platelet serotonin uptake were found in mania. Some studies demonstrated higher platelet serotonin concentration and platelet serotonin uptake in manic patients than in healthy controls, although correlation between these two parameters was not found [Saxena et al., 1999].

Although low platelet MAO activity has been associated with high impulsivity, disinhibition and excessive risk-taking behavior [Verkes et al., 1998], which are often observed in mania, our present findings as well as some other studies [Takahashi, 1977] found no differences in platelet MAO activity. As reduced platelet MAO activity was observed in healthy male smokers in comparison to non-smokers [Berlin and Anthenelli, 2001; Pivac et al., 2006a] and since a high proportion of patients in our study were smokers, our results might suggest that the effect of smoking was counteracted by the diagnosis.

The present findings also showed that patients with mania, unrelated to the presence of psychotic symptoms, have reduced values of serum cholesterol and LDL, but unaltered TG and HDL levels, compared to healthy persons. These findings are in line with reports on the cholesterol status in patients with a single manic [Pae et al., 2004], mixed [Cassidy and Carroll, 2002], or pure manic [Ghaemi et al., 2000; Cassidy and Carroll, 2002; Atmaca et al., 2002a] episode.

Observed altered lipid status in manic patients might be due to the nutritional status, gender, weight loss or physical activity. However, decreased cholesterol levels, observed in our patients, are not related to different body weight, as no differences in BMI among groups were found. Moreover, the hypercholesterolemia among our manic patients is not related to suicidal behavior [Atmaca et al., 2003; Kim and Myint, 2004], since only two patients had history of suicide attempts.

We have found no correlation between high platelet serotonin levels and low cholesterol and LDL levels in patients in mania, and there was no correlation between low platelet serotonin values and low cholesterol levels in suicide attempters [Alvarez et al., 1999]; however it is possible that platelet serotonin and cholesterol levels are negatively correlated only in the presence of hypercholesterolemia [Smith and Betteridge, 1997].

Our findings [present study; Marcinko et al., 2011] demonstrated a lack of significant differences in total serum cholesterol levels between suicidal borderline patients compared to non-suicidal patients with BPD and healthy control subjects. These results are in contrast with our previous [Marcinko et al., 2005; 2007] and numerous other studies, showing an association between low cholesterol levels and suicidal behavior. Namely, it has been suggested that low cholesterol levels may be associated with reduced lipid micro-viscosity of brain-cell-membrane and decreased expression and function of various serotonergic receptors on the membrane surface [Engelberg, 1992]. The resulting inhibition of serotonergic neurotransmission may lead to a poorer suppression of impulsive or suicidal behavior.

However, some authors also found a relation between high cholesterol levels and increased suicidal risk [Brunner et al., 2006], while others observed no association between cholesterol and suicidal behavior [Deisenhammer et al., 2004]. These discrepancies among studies suggest that biologic basis, as well as pharmacologic treatment of BPD, is incompletely studied compared to other psychiatric disorders. Our results showing that cholesterol might not be used to distinguish between suicidal from non-suicidal BPD might be associated with the biologic theory of a poorer response of BPD patients to antidepressants acting via serotonergic system compared to the patients with the other diagnostic categories [Shea et al., 1990].

Moreover, our results demonstrating significantly higher HDRS-17 and BPRS scores in suicidal then in non-suicidal patients could suggest that suicidal behavior is associated with the higher levels of psychopathology. Although, psychotic symptoms in BPRS did not differ between suicidal and non-suicidal BPD patients, seven non-psychotic symptoms in BPRS were significantly higher in suicidal then in non-suicidal patients, suggesting that anxiety, depression, grandiosity, tension, excitement and motor hyperactivity may be associated with development of suicidal behavior.

The results of our study also demonstrated that structured individual psychoanalytic psychotherapy prior to the hospitalization significantly decreased suicidal behavior. Hence in BPD patients, matched for age, BMI, socio-demographic characteristics and serum cholesterol levels, the use of structured individual psychoanalytic psychotherapy prior to the hospitalization elicited a basic distinction between suicidal and non-suicidal groups.

Structured individual psychoanalytic psychotherapy is aimed to enhance patient's personality and to help patient to better cope with BPD symptoms: However, our results suggested that it might be also used in order to better control suicidal symptoms, as well as the symptoms of anxiety, depression, grandiosity, tension, excitement and motor hyperactivity, which were presented more severely in suicidal patients with BPD, in order to prevent suicidal behavior.

Our results demonstrating decreased serum cholesterol levels in suicidal patients in the first episode of psychosis are in agreement with the reports showing lower cholesterol levels in patients with suicidal attempts [Atmaca et al., 2002b; Marcinko et al., 2004; Marcinko et al., 2005]. As already discussed, low cholesterol levels and suicidality might be related to decreased serotonergic neurotransmission [Hawton et al., 1993]. Reduced lipid microviscosity in the brain-cell membrane and consequently decreased expression and function of serotonin receptors on the membrane surface [Engelberg, 1992] could induce alteration in serotonergic activity and function. Inhibited serotonergic neurotransmission may lead to a poorer suppression of impulsive or aggressive behavior, or to a depressive state, triggering a more violent pattern of behavior in susceptible individuals.

Our findings showed that suicidal patients in the first episode of psychosis had lower platelet serotonin concentration than non-suicidal patients. These findings are in line with our previous reports [Muck-Seler et al., 1996; Pivac et al., 1997], demonstrating a relationship between reduced platelet serotonin concentration and suicidal behavior in psychotic and non-psychotic depressed patients. Together, these data support the hypothesis that platelet serotonin concentration, in drug-free patients, might be used as a limited peripheral marker of suicidal behavior, not only in depressed patients, but also in acute psychotic patients. Biological markers are proposed to be associated with a single psychological dysfunction [Muller-Oerlinghausen et al., 2004; Van Praag, 2004], and not with particular diagnostic entities.

In contrast to our results showing low cholesterol levels associated with reduced platelet serotonin concentration in suicidal patients, some studies reported decreased serum cholesterol levels [Vevera et al., 2005] and increased serotonin uptake. The discrepancies between results might be explained by the different protocols used, i.e. baseline data in the first episode of psychosis (present study) vs. data obtained after cholesterol lowering therapy [Vevera et al., 2005; Muldoon et al., 2001]. Platelet serotonin concentration might be also affected by different factors, such as gender, age or season. The effect of gender might be excluded, since our study included only male subjects; while no significant relation between age and platelet serotonin in healthy subjects [Pivac et al., 2001] or in patients in the first episode of psychosis (present study) suggested that the possible effect of age on platelet serotonin content could be neglected. Moreover, since platelet serotonin did not differ significantly when sampled in the different seasons [Jakovljevic et al., 1997], a possible seasonal influence on platelet serotonin may be also ruled out.

Moreover, in line with the studies suggesting an association between depressive symptoms and suicidality in psychotic patients [Aguilar et al., 2003], suicidal patients in our study had more pronounced depressive symptoms, than non-suicidal patients, as shown by higher HDRS-17 scores. However, no significant correlation was found between platelet serotonin and

HDRS-17 scores, or between platelet serotonin and BPRS scores, in our non-suicidal and suicidal patients.

In another study [present results; Muck-Seler et al., 2011], we evaluated the association between the basal lipid profile and clinical response to antidepressants paroxetine or tianeptine in non-suicidal female patients diagnosed with depression. Our results demonstrated higher baseline cholesterol levels in nonresponders then in responders to 4 weeks' treatment with paroxetine. Elevated baseline cholesterol levels have been also found in nonresponders to fluoxetine treatment [Sonawalla et al., 2002]. Together these data suggest that lower serum lipid levels might indicate a better response to selective serotonin reuptake inhibitors, such as paroxetine or fluoxetine.

However, although lipid values detected in our patients were higher than the recommended values for the lipid levels, they were not significantly different from the levels found in healthy women [Sagud et al., 2007]. These findings show that our female subjects (both depressed and healthy) have increased lipid levels. Responders and nonresponders to paroxetine in our study did not differ in age and were without cardiovascular or cerebrovascular cormobidities [Bella et al., 2010], which might influence treatment response [Papakostas et al., 2004a]. The treatment resistance in patients with higher cholesterol values might be due to alterations in serotonergic function. Namely, patients with both depression and hypercholesterolemia had an attenuated prolactin and cortisol response to DL-fenfluramine [Papakostas et al., 2004b], while healthy persons with metabolic syndrome had blunted prolactin response to citalopram [Muldoon et al., 2006]. In this respect, there is evidence that paroxetine treatment may be associated with increased LDL-C and cholesterol levels [Kim and Yu, 2005]. In contrast to paroxetine treatment, the response to tianeptine was not associated with alterations in baseline lipid levels. To the best of our knowledge, these findings were the only ones evaluating the association between response to tianeptine and baseline lipid levels.

Our results demonstrating higher levels of serum cholesterol, HDL-C and TG, and lower levels of LDL-C in female subjects, when compared to male subjects, are in line with other findings, which reported gender-related differences in the lipid profile [Regitz-Zagrosek et al., 2007], and might be explained by the influence of sex hormones, such as estrogen. However, higher serum cholesterol levels with the increase in HDL-C and decrease in LDL-C levels were observed also in the postmenopausal female subjects [Regitz-Zagrosek et al., 2007]. Since the average age of the subjects in our study was about 77 years, all female subjects were already in the postmenopausal stage, so the effects of estrogen on lipid levels is excluded. In these female subjects the lack of cholesterol was related with the altered ratio between HDL-C and LDL-C levels. In line with our results, higher TG levels are found to be the higher risk factor for developing cardiovascular diseases and diabetes in female, then in male subjects [Wilson et al., 1998].

In the present study serum cholesterol levels were significantly associated with the 1997A/G polymorphism of the 5-HT1B receptor gene, in male, but not in the female subjects. Namely, male carriers of the AG genotype had significantly higher serum cholesterol levels, when compared with the male carriers of AA and GG genotypes. However, due to small number of subjects carrying GG genotype, only significant differences in cholesterol levels were found between male carriers of AG and AA genotypes. On the other hand, no association between lipid levels and different genotypes of 5-HT2A and 5-HT2C receptor gene variants was observed, both in male and in female subjects.

Serotonin and serotonergic receptors, including serotonergic 5-HT1B, 5-HT2A and 5-HT2C receptors, play an important role in regulating the food intake, appetite and body weight [Leibowitz and Alexander, 1998]. For instance, serotonin and serotonin agonists have been found to decrease the appetite and BMI [Garfield and Heisler, 2009]. Several studies reported the association of different polymorphisms in 5-HT1B [Levitan et al., 2001], 5-HT2A [Rosmond et al. 2002; Kring et al., 2009] and 5-HT2C [Kring et al., 2009; Vimaleswaran et al., 2010] receptor genes with eating disorders and BMI.

Some studies suggest the association of 5-HT1B receptors with regulation of food intake and body weight [Halford et al., 2007]. Namely, 5-HT1B receptor knock-out mice were found to have increased body weight, although they were not obese [Bouwknecht et al., 2001]. Moreover, the infusion of 5-HT1B receptor agonists directly into the pons has been shown to result in the lower food intake [Lee et al., 1998]. It has been also demonstrated that 5-HT1B receptor activation decreases the synthesis of neuropeptide Y, which stimulates lateral core of hypothalamus, where the feeding center is located. In vitro study of Svenningsson et al. (2006) showed that 5-HT1B receptor co-localize and interact on the cell surface with p11 protein. Lower expression of p11 in the brain has been demonstrated in animal models of depression, as well as in depressive patients, while the increased expression of p11 and higher 5-HT1B receptor function has been observed in the brain of the rats following treatment with antidepressants. Moreover, p11 knock-out mice demonstrated depression-like phenotype and weaker response to 5-HT1B receptor agonists and antidepressants [Svenningsson et al., 2006].

Hence, studies regarding the role of 5-HT1B receptor in regulating the food intake [Lee et al., 1998] and weight [Bouwknecht et al., 2001] were mostly performed on animals, and there is very small amount of data available on the association of human 5-HT1B receptor gene variants and nutrition, most of it obtained in the studies investigating the genetic basis of bulimia [Levitan et al., 2001]. In a study on patients with bulimia, higher BMI was found in GG genotype carriers and lower BMI in CC genotype carriers of 861G/C polymorphism in 5-HT1B receptor gene [Levitan et al., 2001]. On the other hand, the 861G/C polymorphism in 5-HT1B receptor gene has been associated with the development of different neuropsychiatric disorders. Namely, allele 861G has been associated with the attention deficit hyperactivity disorder (ADHD) and antisocial behavior, while the 861C allele has been associated with the development of alcoholism and drug addiction, as well as depression [Smoller et al., 2006; Lee et al., 1998].

A number of studies also reported associations of 5-HT2A receptor gene polymorphisms and different neuropsychiatric disorders, including schizophrenia [Abdolmaleky et al., 2004; Williams et al., 1997], suicide [Videtic et al., 2006], panic disorder [Rothe et al., 2004], alcoholism [Nakamura et al., 1999] and Alzheimer's disease [Nacmias et al., 2001], however the results of these studies were very inconsistent. In addition, several studies demonstrated the association between the specific 5-HT2A receptor gene variant and therapeutic response to rispreridon [Yamanouchi et al., 2003], clozapine [Harvey et al., 2003] or antidepressant [McMahon et al., 2006] treatment.

Our findings of no association between lipid levels and different genotypes of 5-HT2A receptor gene are in line with the results of several studies demonstrating that, although there were significant differences in the cholesterol and TG levels between subjects with normal and subjects with increased body weight, these differences were not associated with different genotypes of A-1438G polymorphism in 5-HT2A receptor gene [Ying et al., 2009; Rosmond et al., 2002]. On the other hand, Kring et al. (2009) found the association of allele A with higher levels of cholesterol, but not with levels of TG and HDL-C in obese subjects [Kring et al., 2009]. Among subjects with normal body weight, lower levels of serum cholesterol and HDL-C have been observed in CC genotype carriers, when compared to carriers of other variants of T102C polymorphism in the 5-HT2A receptor gene [Choi et al., 2005]. These discrepancies in the results might be due to differences in the age of the subjects or ethnic differences in the distribution of alleles, as allele C is more frequently found in Caucasian then in Mongoloid subjects [Choi et al., 2005]. Moreover, Aubert et al. (2000) reported that the 5-HT2A receptor gene variants are associated with the energy intake in the overweighed subjects, while the association of 5-HT2A receptor gene and anorexia nervosa has been often investigated [Kipman et al., 2002].

It has been suggested that increased 5-HT2C receptor activity induces the synthesis of pro-opiomelanocortin, which inhibits the center for feeding, located in the lateral part of hypothalamus, resulting in decreased appetite and food intake, while the deficits in this receptor gene seem to be directly associated with obesity [Lam et al., 2010; Leysen, 2004; Nonogaki et al., 1998; Tecott et al., 1995]. In studies investigating the 759C/T polymorphism of the 5-HT2C receptor gene, C allele has been associated with higher incidence of overweight and higher BMI in patients with mental disorders, but not in healthy subjects with increased BMI [Kring et al., 2009; Miller, 2005; Olajossy-Hilkesberger et al., 2006; Chagnon, 2006; Vimaleswaran et al., 2010]. Since it has been observed that genetic and pharmacological inhibition of 5-HT2C receptor increases the food intake and weight gain [Aloyo et al., 2009; Schreiber and de Vry, 2002; Bonhaus et al., 1997], 5-HT2C receptor selective agonists, such as lorcaserin and m-clorphenilpiperazin, are currently evaluated in the clinical studies for the treatment of obesity [Halford et al., 2007; Bray, 2008; Heisler et al., 2003; Bays, 2009; Lam et al., 2008]. Hence, 5-HT2C receptor has been one of the most important targets for developing new therapeutic approaches in the treatment of eating disorders [Bickerdike et al., 1999]. However, although these findings suggest that lower activity or the absence of 5-HT2C receptor, results in higher food intake and obesity [Lam et al., 2010; Leysen, 2004; Nonogaki et al., 1998; Tecott et al., 1995), in our study we observed no association between lipid levels and different genotypes or alleles of T-759C polymorphism in the 5-HT2C receptor gene.

CONCLUSION

This manuscript summarized the results of our present and previous studies investigating the serum lipid levels and their possible association with different parameters of serotonergic system (platelet serotonin content, platelet MAO activity or 5-HT1B, 5-HT2A and 5-HT2C receptor gene polymorphisms) in healthy subjects and in patients with various neuropsychiatric disorders, including Alzheimer's disease, major depression, bipolar disorder and psychotic mania, as well as their possible association with treatment response to antidepressants.

Our results demonstrated reduction in serum lipid levels in patients with Alzheimer's disease as well as the association between serum cholesterol and LDL-C levels with severity of the disease. The observed positive association between low serum cholesterol and LDL-C levels with cognitive decline during the progress of Alzheimer's disease suggests that increased lipid levels could play the protective role in develop of Alzheimer's disease.

Moreover, our data showed an inverse relationship between HDL-C and TG levels in patients with mood disorders, particularly in those with bipolar disorder (whether in a manic or a depressive phase). Namely, lower HDL-C values were found in patients in depressive and manic phase of bipolar disorder and major depression, and lower cholesterol levels were found in suicidal psychotic patients, while higher TG levels were found in patients with BP than in control subjects. The results imply that low HDL-C levels and high atherogenic index could be hallmark of affective disorders. However, further studies are needed in order to investigate whether low HDL-C levels and a high atherogenic index contribute to a vulnerability to develop affective disorders, or HDL-C levels decreased during the course of mood disorders. In addition, the observed changes in lipid profile suggest also that patients with BP and MDD are at higher risk for the development of coronary heart disease.

In our study we observed the increase in platelet serotonin concentrations and decrease in serum cholesterol and LDL-C levels which could be the characteristic features of psychotic subtype in patients in a manic phase of BP. Our findings also supported the hypothesis that platelet serotonin concentration might be used as a peripheral biomarker for the psychotic states. Namely, increased platelet serotonin, found across different diagnoses, suggests that psychotic subtypes of the different diagnostic entities might share similar biochemical abnormalities.

The findings of our study demonstrated no significant association between serum lipid levels and response to tianeptine. The preliminary results with paroxetine might indicate that patients with depression and higher than normal baseline cholesterol, TG, and LDL-C levels may be suitable candidates for the initiation or addition of the antidepressant with the mechanism of action different from paroxetine.

Moreover, the observed association of serum cholesterol levels with 5-HT1B receptor gene polymorphism in healthy subjects is in line with results demonstrating the interaction of lipids with serotonergic system.

In conclusion, the results of our studies reviewed here support the hypothesis of an association between altered lipid homeostasis and development and progress of different neuropsychiatric disorders, as well as treatment response. Moreover, our findings demonstrate the relationship between serum lipid levels and serotonergic system in healthy subjects, as well as in neuropsychiatric patients. However, further investigations of lipid metabolism and serotonergic system are needed in order to better understand their role in the neurobiology of these disorders and to develop better treatment interventions for neuropsychiatric patients.

ACKNOWLEDGMENTS

Thanks are due to the psychiatric staff of the University Hospital Center Zagreb, Clinics for Psychiatry Vrapce, Psychiatric Hospital Sveti Ivan, Jankomir and Institute for Medical Research and Occupational Health, Zagreb, Croatia. This work was supported by the Croatian Ministry of Science, Education and Sport, grants numbers 098-0982522-2455, 098-0922522-2457 and 108-1080037-0323.

REFERENCES

Abad-Rodriguez, J; Ledesma, MD; Craessaerts, K; Perga, S; Medina, M; Delacourte, A; Dingwall, C; De Strooper, B; Dotti, CG. Neuronal membrane cholesterol loss enhances amyloid peptide generation. *J Cell Biol,* 2004, 167, 953-960.

Abdolmaleky, HM; Faraone, SV; Glatt, SJ; Tsuang, MT. Meta-analysis of association between the T102C polymorphism of the 5HT2a receptor gene and schizophrenia. *Schizophr Res,* 2004, 67; 53-62.

Adibhatla, RM; Hatcher, JF. Altered lipid metabolism in brain injury and disorders. *Subcell Biochem,* 2008, 49, 241-268.

Agargün, MY; Algün, E; Sekeroğlu, R; Kara, H; Tarakçioğlu, M. Low cholesterol level in patients with panic disorder: the association with major depression. *J Affect Disord,* 1998, 50, 29-32.

Agargun, MY; Ozer, OA; Kara, H; Sekeroglu, R; Selvi, Y; Eryonucu, B. Serum lipid levels in patients with dissociative disorder. *Am J Psychiatry,* 2004, 161, 2121-2123.

Aguilar, EJ; Leal, C; Acosta, FJ; Cejas, MR; Fernández, L; Gracia, R. A psychopathological study of a group of schizophrenic patients after attempting suicide. Are there two different clinical subtypes? *Eur Psychiatry,* 2003, 18, 190-192.

Allen, JA; Halverson-Tamboli, RA; Rasenick, MM. Lipid raft microdomains and neurotransmitter signaling. *Nat Rev Neurosci,* 2007, 8, 128-140.

Almeida-Montes, LG; Valles-Sanchez, V; Moreno-Aguilar, J; Chavez-Balderas, RA; García-Marín, JA; Cortés Sotres, JF; Hheinze-Martin, G. Relation of serum cholesterol, lipid, serotonin and tryptophan levels to severity of depression and to suicide attempts. *J Psychiatry Neurosci,* 2000, 25, 371-377.

Alvarez, JC; Cremniter, D; Gluck, N; Quintin, P; Leboyer, M; Berlin, I; Therond, P; Spreux-Varoquaux, O. Low serum cholesterol in violent but not in non-violent suicide attempters. *Psychiatry Res,* 2000, 95, 103-108.

Alvarez, JC; Cremniter, D; Lesieur, P; Gregoire, A; Gilton, A; Macquin-Mavier, I; Jarreau, C; Spreux-Varoquaux, O. Low blood cholesterol and low platelet serotonin levels in violent suicide attempters. *Biol Psychiatry,* 1999, 45, 1066-1069.

Aloyo, VJ; Berg, KA; Spampinato, U; Clarke, WP; Harvey, JA. Current status of inverse agonism at serotonin2A (5-HT2A) and 5-HT2C receptors. *Pharmacol Ther,* 2009, 121, 160-173.

American Psychiatric Association. *Diagnostic and Statistical Manual of Mental Disorders.* IV Edition. American Psychiatric Press, Washington, DC, 2000.

Anderson, RWG; Jacobson, K. A role for lipid shells in targeting proteins to caveolae, rafts, and other lipid domains. *Science,* 2002, 296, 1821–1825.

Atmaca, M; Kuloglu, M; Tezcan, E; Ustundag, B. Serum leptin and triglyceride levels in patients on treatment with atypical antipsychotics. *J Clin Psychiatry,* 2003, 64, 598-604.

Atmaca, M; Kuloglu, M; Tezcan, E; Ustundag, B. Serum leptin and cholesterol values in violent and non-violent suicide attempters. *Psychiatry Res,* 2008, 158, 87-91.

Atmaca, M; Kuloglu, M; Tezcan, E; Ustundag, B; Bayik, Y. Serum leptin and cholesterol levels in patients with bipolar disorder. *Neuropsychobiology,* 2002a, 46, 176-179.

Atmaca, M; Kuloglu, M; Tezcan, E; Ustundag, B; Gecici, O; Firidin, B. Serum leptin and cholesterol values in suicide attempters. *Neuropsychobiology,* 2002b, 45, 124-127.

Aubert, R; Betoulle, D; Herbeth, B; Siest, G; Fumeron, F. 5-HT2A receptor gene polymorphism is associated with food and alcohol intake in obese people. *Int J Obes Relat Metab Disord*, 2000; 24, 920-924.

Baier, CJ; Barrantes, FJ. Sphingolipids are necessary for nicotinic acetylcholine receptor export in the early secretory pathway. *J Neurochem,* 2007, 101, 1072–1084.

Bays, HE; Lorcaserin and adiposopathy: 5-HT2c agonism as a treatment for 'sick fat' and metabolic disease. *Expert Rev Cardiovasc Ther,* 2009, 7, 1429-1445.

Bajwa, WK; Asnis, GM; Sanderson, WC; Irfan, A; van Praag, HM. High cholesterol levels in patients with panic disorder. *Am J Psychiatry,* 1992, 149, 376-378.

Beasley, CL; Honer, WG; Bergmann, K; Falkai, P, Lütjohann, D; Bayer, TA. Reductions in cholesterol and synaptic markers in association cortex in mood disorders. *Bipolar Disord,* 2005, 7, 449-455.

Bella, R; Pennisi, G; Cantone, M; Palermo, F; Pennisi, M; Lanza, G; Zappia, M; Paolucci, S. Clinical presentation and outcome of geriatric depression in subcortical ischemic vascular disease. Gerontology, 2010, 56, 298-302.

Berlin, I; Anthenelli, RM. Monoamine oxidases and tobacco smoking. *Int J Neuropsychopharmacol,* 2001, 4, 33-42.

Berridge, MJ. Inositol trisphosphate and diacylglycerol as second messengers. *Biochem J,* 1984, 220, 345–630.

Bickerdike, MJ; Vickers, SP; Dourish, CT. 5-HT2C receptor modulation and the treatment of obesity. *Diabetes Obes Metab,* 1999, 1, 207-214.

Bilici, M; Efe, H; Köroğlu, MA; Uydu, HA; Bekaroğlu, M; Değer, O. Antioxidative enzyme activities and lipid peroxidation in major depression: alterations by antidepressant treatments. *J Affect Disord,* 2001, 64, 43-51.

Bocchetta, A; Chillotti, C; Carboni, G; Oi, A; Ponti, M, Del Zompo, M. Association of personal and familial suicide risk with low serum cholesterol concentration in male lithium patients. *Acta Psychiatr Scand,* 2001, 104, 37-41.

Bonarek, M; Barberger-Gateau, P; Letenneur, L; Deschamps, V; Iron, A; Dubroca, B; Dartigues, JF. Relationships between cholesterol, apolipoprotein E polymorphism and dementia: a cross-sectional analysis from the PAQUID study. *Neuroepidemiology*, 2000, 19, 141-148.

Bonhaus, DW; Weinhardt, KK; Taylor, M; DeSouza, A; McNeeley, PM; Szczepanski, K; Fontana, DJ; Trinh, J; Rocha, CL; Dawson, MW, Flippin, LA; Eglen, RM. RS-102221: a novel high affinity and selective, 5-HT2C receptor antagonist. *Neuropharmacology,* 1997, 36, 621-629.

Boston, PF; Dursun, SM, Reveley, MA. Cholesterol and mental disorder. *Br J Psychiatry,* 1996, 169, 682-689.

Bouwknecht, JA; van der Gugten, J; Hijzen, TH; Maes, RA; Hen, R; Olivier, B. Male and female 5-HT(1B) receptor knockout mice have higher body weights than wildtypes. *Physiol Behav,* 2001, 74, 507-516.

Bray, MS. Implications of gene-behavior interactions: prevention and intervention for obesity. *Obesity* (Silver Spring), 2008, 16, (Suppl 3), S72-78.

Brown, RA; Giggey, PP; Dennis, KE; Waldstein, SR. Depression and lipoprotein lipids in healthy, postmenopausal women; the moderating effects of hormone replacement therapy. *J Psychosom Res,* 2004, 57; 171-176.

Brown, SL; Salive, ME; Harris, TB; Simonsick, EM; Guralnik, JM; Kohout, FJ. Low cholesterol concentrations and severe depressive symptoms in elderly people. *BMJ,* 1994, 308, 1328-1332.

Brunner, J; Bronisch, T; Pfister, H; Jacobi, F; Höfler, M; Wittchen, HU. High cholesterol, triglycerides, and body-mass index in suicide attempters. *Arch Suicide Res,* 2006, 10, 1-9.

Burger, K; Gimpl, G; Fahrenholz, F: Regulation of receptor function by cholesterol. *Cell Mol Life Sci,* 2000, 57, 1577–1592.

Buydens-Branchey, L; Branchey, M; Hudson, J; Fergeson, P. Low HDL cholesterol, aggression and altered central serotonergic activity. *Psychiatry Res,* 2000, 93, 93-102.

Caballero, J; Nahata, M. Do statins slow down Alzheimer's disease? A review. *J Clin Pharm Ther,* 2004, 29, 209-213.

Cadeddu, G; Fioravanti, P; Antonicelli, R; Gasparrini, PM; Gaetti, R. Relationship between cholesterol levels and depression in the elderly. *Minerva Med,* 1995, 86, 251–256.

Cagnin, A; Zambon, A; Zarantonello, G; Vianello, D; Marchiori, M; Mercurio, D; Miccichè, F; Ermani, M; Leon, A; Battistin, L. Serum lipoprotein profile and APOE genotype in Alzheimer's disease. *J Neural Transm Suppl,* 2007, 72, 175-179.

Callréus, T; Agerskov Andersen, U; Hallas, J, Andersen, M. Cardiovascular drugs and the risk of suicide: a nested case-control study. *Eur J Clin Pharmacol,* 2007, 63, 591-596.

Canevari, L; Clark, JB. Alzheimer's disease and cholesterol: the fat connection. *Neurochem Res,* 2007, 32, 739-750.

Cassidy, F; Carroll, BJ. Hypocholesterolemia during mixed manic episodes. *Eur Arch Psychiatry Clin Neurosci,* 2002, 252, 110-114.

Chakrabarti, N; Sinha, VK. A study of serum lipid profile and serum apolipoproteins A1 and B in Indian male violent criminal offenders. *Crim Behav Ment Health,* 2006, 16, 177-182.

Chagnon, YC. Susceptibility genes for the side effect of antipsychotics on body weight and obesity. *Curr Drug Targets,* 2006, 7, 1681-1695.

Charney, DS; Redmond, DE Jr. Neurobiological mechanisms in human anxiety. Evidence supporting central noradrenergic hyperactivity. *Neuropharmacology,* 1983, 22, 1531-1536.

Chauhan, NB. Membrane dynamics, cholesterol homeostasis, and Alzheimer's disease. *J Lipid Res,* 2003, 44, 2019-2029.

Chen, CC; Lu, FH; Wu, JS; Chang, CJ. Correlation between serum lipid concentrations and psychological distress. *Psychiatry Res,* 2001, 102, 153-162.

Choi, JH; Zhang, SY; Park, KW; Cho, YS; Oh, BH; Lee, MM; Park, YB; Kim, HS. The association between the T102C polymorphism of the HTR2A serotonin receptor gene and HDL cholesterol level in Koreans. *J Biochem Mol Biol,* 2005, 38, 238-242.

Cleare, AJ; Murray, RM; O'Keane, V. Assessment of serotonergic function in major depression using d-fenfluramine: relation to clinical variables and antidepressant response. *Biol Psychiatry,* 1998, 44, 555-561

Coccaro, EF; Kavoussi, RJ; Cooper, TB; Hauger, RL. Hormonal responses to d- and d,l-fenfluramine in healthy human subjects. *Neuropsychopharmacology.*1996, 15, 595-607.

Cohen, RA; Zitnay, KM; Haudenschild, CC; Cunningham, LD. Loss of selective endothelial cell vasoactive functions caused by hypercholesterolemia in pig coronary arteries. *Circ Res,* 1988, 63, 903-910.

Conklin, SM; Stanford, MS. Premeditated aggression is associated with serum cholesterol in abstinent drug and alcohol dependent men. *Psychiatry Res,* 2008, 157, 283-287.

Coto, E; Reguero, JR; Alvarez, V; Morales, B; Batalla, A; González, P; Martín, M; García-Castro, M; Iglesias-Cubero, G; Cortina, A. 5-Hydroxytryptamine 5-HT2A receptor and 5-hydroxytryptamine transporter polymorphisms in acute myocardial infarction. *Clin Sci* (Lond), 2003, 104, 241-245.

Cowen, PJ. Serotonin receptor subtypes in depression: evidence from studies in neuroendocrine regulation. *Clin Neuropharmacol,* 1993, 16, (Suppl 3), 6-18.

Cummings, JL; Mega, M; Gray, K; Rosenberg-Thompson, S; Carusi, DA; Gornbein, J. The Neuropsychiatric Inventory: comprehensive assessment of psychopathology in dementia. *Neurology,* 1994, 44, 2308-2314.

Deisenhammer, EA; Kramer-Reinstadler, K; Liensberger, D; Kemmler, G; Hinterhuber, H; Fleischhacker, WW. No evidence for an association between serum cholesterol and the course of depression and suicidality. *Psychiatry Res,* 2004, 121, 253-261.

Diaz-Sastre, C; Baca-Garcia, E; Perez-Rodriguez, MM; Garcia-Resa, E; Ceverino, A; Saiz-Ruiz, J; Oquendo, MA; de Leon, J. Low plasma cholesterol levels in suicidal males: a gender- and body mass index-matched case-control study of suicide attempters and nonattempters. *Prog Neuropsychopharmacol Biol Psychiatry,* 2007, 31, 901-905.

Diebold K; Michel, G; Schweizer, J; Diebold-Dörsam, M; Fiehn, W; Kohl, B. Are psychoactive-drug-induced changes in plasma lipid and lipoprotein levels of significance for clinical remission in psychiatric disorders? *Pharmacopsychiatry*, 1998, 31, 60-67.

Eckert, GP; Wood, WG; Muller, WE. Statins: drugs for Alzheimer's disease? *J Neural Transm,* 2005, 112, 1057-1071.

Edgar, PF; Hooper, AJ; Poa, NR; Burnett, JR. Violent behavior associated with hypocholesterolemia due to a novel APOB gene mutation. *Mol Psychiatry,* 2007, 12, 258-263.

Ellison, LF; Morrison, HI. Low serum cholesterol concentration and risk of suicide. *Epidemiology,* 2001, 12, 168-172.

Engelberg, H. Low serum cholesterol and suicide. Lancet, 1992, 339, 727-729.

Engström, G; Alsén, M; Regnéll, G; Träskman-Bendz, L. Serum lipids in suicide attempters. *Suicide Life Threat Behav,* 1995, 25, 393-400.

Fan, J; Watanabe, T. Cholesterol-fed and transgenic rabbit models for the study of atherosclerosis. *J Atheroscler Thromb*, 2000, 7, 26-32.

Fantini, J; Barrantes, FJ. Sphingolipid/cholesterol regulation of neurotransmitter receptor conformation and function. *Biochim Biophys Acta,* 2009, 1788, 2345-2361.

Fava, M. Depression with anger attacks. *J Clin Psychiatry,* 1998, 59, Suppl 18, 18-22.

Fava, M; Abraham, M; Pava, J; Shuster, J; Rosenbaum, J. Cardiovascular risk factors in depression. The role of anxiety and anger. *Psychosomatics,* 1996, 37, 31-37.

Fava, M; Rosenbaum, JF. Anger attacks in depression. *Depress Anxiety,* 1998, 8 Suppl 1, 59-63.

Fava, M; Vuolo, RD; Wright, EC; Nierenberg, AA; Alpert, JE; Rosenbaum, JF. Fenfluramine challenge in unipolar depression with and without anger attacks. *Psychiatry Res,* 2000, 94, 9-18.

Fiedorowicz, JG; Coryell, WH. Cholesterol and suicide attempts: a prospective study of depressed inpatients. *Psychiatry Res,* 2007, 152, 11-20.

Fiedorowicz, JG; Palagummi, NM; Forman-Hoffman, VL; Miller, DD; Haynes, WG. Elevated prevalence of obesity, metabolic syndrome, and cardiovascular risk factors in bipolar disorder. *Ann Clin Psychiatry,* 2008, 20, 131-137.

First, MB; Spitzer, RL; Gibbon, M; Williams, JB. Clinical Interview for Axis I DSM-IV Disorders. *Structured Clinical Interview for Axis I DSM-IV Disorders*. New York State Psychiatric Institute, New York, NY, 1995.

Fischer, P; Gruenblatt, E; Pietschmann, P; Tragl, KH. Serotonin transporter polymorphism and LDL-cholesterol. *Mol Psychiatry,* 2006, 11, 707-709.

Folstein, MF; Folstein, SE; McHugh, PR. "Mini-mental state". A practical method for grading the cognitive state of patients for the clinician. *J Psychiatr Res,* 1975, 12, 189-198.

Fontenot, MB; Kaplan, JR; Shively, CA; Manuck, SB; Mann, JJ. Cholesterol, serotonin, and behavior in young monkeys. *Ann N Y Acad Sci,* 1996, 794, 352-354.

Franceschini, G. Epidemiologic evidence for high-density lipoprotein cholesterol as a risk factor for coronary artery disease. *Am J Cardiol,* 2001, 88, 9N-13N.

Freedman, DS; Byers, T; Barrett, DH; Stroup, NE; Eaker, E; Monroe-Blum, H. Plasma lipid levels and psychologic characteristics in men. *Am J Epidemiol,* 1995, 141, 507–517.

Frick, MH; Elo, O; Haapa, K; Heinonen, OP; Heinsalmi, P; Helo, P; Huttunen, JK; Kaitaniemi, P; Koskinen, P; Manninen, V. et al. Helsinki Heart Study: primary-prevention trial with gemfibrozil in middle-aged men with dyslipidemia. Safety of treatment, changes in risk factors, and incidence of coronary heart disease. *N Engl J Med,* 1987, 317, 1237-1245.

Frikke-Schmidt, R; Nordestgaard, BG; Agerholm-Larsen, B; Schnohr, P; Tybjaerg-Hansen, A. Context-dependent and invariant associations between lipids, lipoproteins, and apolipoproteins and apolipoprotein E genotype. *J Lipid Res,* 2000, 41, 1812-1822.

Fumeron, F; Betoulle, D; Nicaud, V; Evans, A; Kee, F; Ruidavets, JB; Arveiler, D; Luc, G; Cambien, F. Serotonin transporter gene polymorphism and myocardial infarction: Etude Cas-Témoins de l'Infarctus du Myocarde (ECTIM). *Circulation,* 2002, 105, 2943-2945.

Gabriel, A. Changes in plasma cholesterol in mood disorder patients: does treatment make a difference? *J Affect Disord*, 2007, 99, 273-278.

Gallerani, M; Manfredini, R; Caracciolo, S; Scapoli, C; Molinari, S; Fersini, C. Serum cholesterol concentrations in parasuicide. *BMJ,* 1995, 310, 1632-1636.

Garfield, AS; Heisler, LK. Pharmacological targeting of the serotonergic system for the treatment of obesity. *J Physiol,* 2009, 587, 49-60.

Garland, MR; Hallahan, B; McNamara, M; Carney, PA; Grimes, H; Hibbeln, JR; Harkin, A; Conroy, RM. Lipids and essential fatty acids in patients presenting with self-harm. *Br J Psychiatry,* 2007, 190, 112-117.

Garland, M; Hickey, D; Corvin, A, Golden, J, Fitzpatrick, P; Cunningham, S; Walsh, N. Total serum cholesterol in relation to psychological correlates in parasuicide. *Br J Psychiatry,* 2000, 177, 77-83.

Ghaemi, SM; Shields, GS; Hegarty, JD; Goodwin, FK. Cholesterol levels in mood disorders: High or low? *Bipolar Disord,* 2000, 2, 60–64.

Glueck, CJ; Tieger, M; Kunkel, R; Hamer, T; Tracy, T; Speirs, J. Hypocholesterolemia and affective disorders. *Am J Med Sci,* 1994, 308, 218-225.

Golier, JA; Marzuk, PM; Leon, AC; Weiner, C; Tardiff, K. Low serum cholesterol level and attempted suicide. *Am J Psychiatry,* 1995, 152, 419-423.

Golomb, BA. Cholesterol and violence: is there a connection? *Ann Intern Med,* 1998, 128, 478-487.

Golomb, BA; Stattin, H; Mednick, S. Low cholesterol and violent crime. *J Psychiatr Res,* 2000, 34, 301-309.

Goodenowe, DB; Cook, LL; Liu, J; Lu Y; Jayasinghe, DA; Ahiahonu, PW; Heath, D; Yamazaki, Y; Flax, J; Krenitsky, KF, Sparks, DL; Lerner, A; Friedland, RP; Kudo, T; Kamino, K; Morihara, T; Takeda, M; Wood, PL. Peripheral ethanolamine plasmalogen deficiency: a logical causative factor in Alzheimer's disease and dementia. *J Lipid Res,* 2007, 48, 2485–2498.

Gorio, A. Ganglioside enhancement of neuronal differentiation, plasticity, and repair. *CRC Crit Rev Clin Neurobiol*, 1986, 2, 241–296.

Grossi, E; Massini, G; Buscema, M; Savarè, R; Maurelli, G. Two different Alzheimer diseases in men and women: clues from advanced neural networks and artificial intelligence. *Gend Med,* 2005, 2, 106-117.

Hakomori, S. The glycosynapse. *Proc Natl Acad Sci USA*, 2002, 99, 225–232.

Halford, JC; Harrold, JA; Boyland, EJ; Lawton, CL; Blundell, JE. Serotonergic drugs: effects on appetite expression and use for the treatment of obesity. *Drugs,* 2007, 67, 27-55.

Hamilton, M. A rating scale for depression. *J Neurol Neurosurg Psychiatry,* 1960, 23, 56-62.

Hartmann, T; Kuchenbecker, J; Grimm, MO. Alzheimer's disease: the lipid connection. *J Neurochem,* 2007, 103, (Suppl 1), 159-170.

Harvey, L; Reid, RE; Ma, C; Knight, PJ; Pfeifer, TA; Grigliatti, TA. Human genetic variations in the 5HT2A receptor: a single nucleotide polymorphism identified with altered response to clozapine. *Pharmacogenetics,* 2003, 13, 107-118.

Hawton, K; Fagg, J; Platt, S; Hawkins, M. Factors associated with suicide after parasuicide in young people. *BMJ,* 1993, 306, 1641-1644.

Hayward, C; Taylor, CB; Roth, WT; King, R; Agras, WS. Plasma lipid levels in patients with panic disorder or agoraphobia. *Am J Psychiatry,* 1989, 146; 917-919.

Heisler, LK; Cowley, M; Kishi, T; Tecott, LH; Fan, W; Low, MJ; Smart, JL; Rubinstein, M; Tatro, JB; Zigman, JM; Cone, RD; Elmquist, JK. Central serotonin and melanocortin pathways regulating energy homeostasis. *Ann N Y Acad Sci,* 2003, 994, 169-174.

Heron, DS; Shinitzky, M; Hershkowitz, M; Samuel, D. Lipid fluidity markedly modulates the binding of serotonin to mouse brain membranes. *Proc Natl Acad Sci USA*, 1980, 77, 7463-7467.

Herrán, A; Ramírez, ML; Carrera, M; García-Unzueta, MT; Sierra-Biddle, D; Rodríguez-Cabo, B; Ayestarán, A; Hoyuela, F; Vázquez-Barquero, JL. Panic disorder, treatment with selective serotonin reuptake inhibitors, and cholesterol levels. *J Clin Psychopharmacol,* 2006, 26, 538-540.

Heverin, M; Meaney, S; Brafman, A; Shafir, M; Olin, M; Shafaati, M; von Bahr, S; Larsson, L; Lövgren-Sandblom, A; Diczfalusy, U; Parini, P, Feinstein, E; Björkhem, I. Studies on the cholesterol-free mouse: strong activation of LXR-regulated hepatic genes when replacing cholesterol with desmosterol. *Arterioscler Thromb Vasc Biol,* 2007, 27, 2191-2197.

Hibbeln, JR; Umhau, JC; George, DT; Shoaf, SE; Linnoila, M; Salem, N Jr. Plasma total cholesterol concentrations do not predict cerebrospinal fluid neurotransmitter metabolites: implications for the biophysical role of highly unsaturated fatty acids. *Am J Clin Nutr,* 2000, 71, (1 Suppl), 331S-338S.

Hibbeln, JR; Umhau, JC; Linnoila, M; George, DT; Ragan, PW; Shoaf, SE; Vaughan, MR; Rawlings, R; Salem, N Jr. A replication study of violent and nonviolent subjects: cerebrospinal fluid metabolites of serotonin and dopamine are predicted by plasma essential fatty acids. *Biol Psychiatry,* 1998, 44, 243-249.

Hillbrand, M; Waite, BM; Miller, DS; Spitz, RT; Lingswiler, VM. Serum cholesterol concentrations and mood states in violent psychiatric patients: an experience sampling study. *J Behav Med,* 2000, 23, 519-529.

Horsten, M; Wamala, SP; Vingerhoets, A; Orth-Gomer, K. Depressive symptoms, social support, and lipid profile in healthy middle-aged women. *Psychosom Med,* 1997, 59, 521–528.

Hu, J; Zhang, Z; Shen, W-J; Azhar, S. Cellular cholesterol delivery, intracellular processing and utilization for biosynthesis of steroid hormones. *Nutr Metab,* 2010, 7, 47.

Huang, TL. Serum lipid profiles in major depression with clinical subtypes, suicide attempts and episodes. *J Affect Disord,* 2005, 86, 75-79.

Ichikawa, N; Iwabuchi, K; Kurihara, H; Ishii, K; Kobayashi, T; Sasaki, T; Hattori, N; Mizuno, Y; Hozumi, K; Yamada, Y; Arikawa-Hirasawa, E. Binding of laminin-1 to monosialoganglioside GM1 in lipid rafts is crucial for neurite outgrowth. *J Cell Sci,* 2009, 122, 289–299.

Iribarren, C; Reed, DM; Chen, R, Yano, K; Dwyer, JH. Low serum cholesterol and mortality. Which is the cause and which is the effect? *Circulation,* 1995, 92, 2396-2403.

Jakovljevic, M; Muck-Seler, D; Pivac, N; Ljubicic, D; Bujas, M; Dodig, G. Seasonal influence on platelet 5-HT levels in patients with recurrent major depression and schizophrenia. *Biol Psychiatry,* 1997, 41, 1028-1034.

Jick, H; Zornberg, GL; Jick, SS; Seshadri, S; Drachman, DA. Statins and the risk of dementia. *Lancet,* 2000, 356, 1627-1631.

Kagan, BL; Leskin, G; Haas, B; Wilkins, J; Foy, D. Elevated lipid levels in Vietnam veterans with chronic posttraumatic stress disorder. *Biol Psychiatry,* 1999, 45, 374-377.

Kahn, RS; Wetzler, S. m-Chlorophenylpiperazine as a probe of serotonin function. *Biol Psychiatry,* 1991, 30, 1139-1166.

Kaplan, JR; Manuck, SB; Shively, C. The effects of fat and cholesterol on social behavior in monkeys. *Psychosom Med,* 1991, 53, 634-642.

Kaplan, JR; Muldoon, MF; Manuck, SB; Mann, JJ. Assessing the observed relationship between low cholesterol and violence-related mortality. Implications for suicide risk. *Ann N Y Acad Sci,* 1997, 836, 57-80.

Kaplan, JR; Shively, CA; Fontenot, MB; Morgan, TM; Howell, SM; Manuck, SB; Muldoon, MF; Mann, JJ. Demonstration of an association among dietary cholesterol, central serotonergic activity, and social behavior in monkeys. *Psychosom Med,* 1994, 56, 479-484.

Karishma, KK; Herbert, J. Dehydroepiandrosterone (DHEA) stimulates neurogenesis in the hippocampus of the rat, promotes survival of newly formed neurons and prevents corticosterone-induced suppression. *Eur J Neurosci,* 2002, 16, 445-453.

Kawarabayashi, T; Shoji, M. Plasma biomarkers of Alzheimer's disease. *Current Opinion in Psychiatry,* 2008, 21, 260–267.

Kim, EJ; Yu, BH. Increased cholesterol levels after paroxetine treatment in patients with panic disorder. J Clin Psychopharmacol, 2005, 25, 597-599.

Kim, YK; Lee, HJ; Kim, JY; Yoon, DK; Choi, SH; Lee, MS. Low serum cholesterol is correlated to suicidality in a Korean sample. *Acta Psychiatr Scand,* 2002, 105, 141-148.

Kim, YK; Myint, AM. Clinical application of low serum cholesterol as an indicator for suicide risk in major depression. *J Affect Disord,* 2004, 81, 161-166.

Kipman, A; Bruins-Slot, L; Boni, C; Hanoun, N; Adès, J; Blot, P; Hamon, M; Mouren-Siméoni, M; Gorwood, P. 5-HT(2A) gene promoter polymorphism as a modifying rather than a vulnerability factor in anorexia nervosa. *Eur Psychiatry,* 2002, 17, 227-229.

Kivipelto, M; Helkala, EL; Laakso, MP; Hanninen, T; Hallikainen, M; Alhainen, K; Iivonen, S; Mannermaa, A, Tuomilehto, J; Nissinen, A, Soininen, H. Apolipoprotein E epsilon4 allele, elevated midlife total cholesterol level, and high midlife systolic blood pressure are independent risk factors for late-life Alzheimer disease. *Ann Intern Med,* 2002, 137, 149-155.

Koudinov, AR; Koudinova, NV. Cholesterol homeostasis failure as a unifying cause of synaptic degeneration. *J Neurol Sci,* 2005, 229-230, 233-240.

Krajl, M. A rapid microfluorimetric determination of monoamine oxidase. *Biochem Pharmacol,* 1965, 14, 1684-1686.

Kring, SI; Werge, T; Holst, C; Toubro, S; Astrup, A; Hansen, T; Pedersen, O; Sorensen, TI. Polymorphisms of serotonin receptor 2A and 2C genes and COMT in relation to obesity and type 2 diabetes. *PLoS One,* 2009, 4, e6696.

Kuczmierczyk, AR; Barbee, JG; Bologna, NA; Townsend, MH. Serum cholesterol levels in patients with generalized anxiety disorder (GAD) and with GAD and comorbid major depression. *Can J Psychiatry,* 1996, 41, 465-468.

Kunugi, H; Takei, N; Aoki, H; Nanko, S. Low serum cholesterol in suicide attempters. *Biol Psychiatry,* 1997, 41, 196-200.

Kuo, YM; Emmerling, MR; Bisgaier, CL; Essenburg, AD; Lampert, HC; Drumm, D; Roher, AE. Elevated low-density lipoprotein in Alzheimer's disease correlates with brain abeta 1-42 levels. *Biochem Biophys Res Commun,* 1998, 252, 711-715.

Lalovic, A; Levy, E; Canetti, L; Sequeira, A; Montoudis, A; Turecki, G. Fatty acid composition in postmortem brains of people who completed suicide. *J Psychiatry Neurosci,* 2007a, 32, 363-370.

Lalovic, A; Levy, E; Luheshi, G; Canetti, L; Grenier, E; Sequeira, A; Turecki, G. Cholesterol content in brains of suicide completers. *Int J Neuropsychopharmacol,* 2007b, 10, 159-166.

Lalovic, A; Merkens, L; Russell, L; Arsenault-Lapierre, G; Nowaczyk, MJ; Porter, FD; Steiner, RD; Turecki, G. Cholesterol metabolism and suicidality in Smith-Lemli-Opitz syndrome carriers. *Am J Psychiatry,* 2004, 161, 2123-2126.

Lam, DD; Przydzial, MJ; Ridley, SH; Yeo, GS; Rochford, JJ; O'Rahilly, S; Heisler, LK. Serotonin 5-HT2C receptor agonist promotes hypophagia via downstream activation of melanocortin 4 receptors. *Endocrinology,* 2008, 149, 1323-1328.

Lam, DD; Garfield, AS; Marston, OJ; Shaw, J; Heisler, LK. Brain serotonin system in the coordination of food intake and body weight. *Pharmacol Biochem Behav,* 2010, 97, 84-91.

Lamping, KG; Nuno, DW; Chappell, DA; Faraci, FM. Agonist-specific impairment of coronary vascular function in genetically altered, hyperlipidemic mice. *Am J Physiol,* 1999, 276, R1023-1029.

Ledesma, MD; Dotti, CG. The conflicting role of brain cholesterol in Alzheimer's disease: lessons from the brain plasminogen system. *Biochem Soc Symp,* 2005, 129-138.

Lee, HJ; Kim, YK. Serum lipid levels and suicide attempts. *Acta Psychiatr Scand,* 2003, 108, 215-221.

Lee, HZ; Lin, WC; Yeh, FT; Wu, CH. 2-Phenyl-4-quinolone prevents serotonin-induced increases in endothelial permeability to albumin. *Eur J Pharmacol,* 1998, 354, 205-213.

Lehto, SM; Hintikka, J; Niskanen, L; Tolmunen, T; Koivumaa-Honkanen, H; Honkalampi, K; Viinamäki, H. Low HDL cholesterol associates with major depression in a sample with a 7-year history of depressive symptoms. *Prog Neuropsychopharmacol Biol Psychiatry,* 2008, 32, 1557-1561.

Leibowitz, SF, Alexander, JT. Hypothalamic serotonin in control of eating behavior, meal size, and body weight. Biol Psychiatry, 1998, 44, 851-864.

Lesperance, F; Frasure-Smith, N, Talajic, M. Major depression before and after myocardial infarction: its nature and consequences. *Psychosom Med,* 1996, 58, 99-110.

Lesser, GT; Haroutunian, V; Purohit, DP; Schnaider Beeri, M; Schmeidler, J; Honkanen, L; Neufeld, R; Libow, LS. Serum lipids are related to Alzheimer's pathology in nursing home residents. *Dement Geriatr Cogn Disord,* 2009, 27, 42-49.

Lester, D. Serum cholesterol levels and suicide: a meta-analysis. *Suicide Life Threat Behav,* 2002, 32, 333-346.

Levitan, RD; Kaplan, AS; Masellis, M; Basile, VS; Walker, ML; Lipson, N; Siegel, GI; Woodside, DB; Macciardi, FM; Kennedy, SH; Kennedy, JL. Polymorphism of the serotonin 5-HT1B receptor gene (HTR1B) associated with minimum lifetime body mass index in women with bulimia nervosa. *Biol Psychiatry,* 2001, 50, 640-643.

Leysen, JE. 5-HT2 receptors. Current Drug Targets – CNS Neurological Disorders, 2004, 1 11-26.

Li, G; Shofer, JB; Kukull, WA; Peskind, ER; Tsuang, DW; Breitner, JC; McCormick, W; Bowen, JD; Teri, L; Schellenberg, GD; Larson, EB. Serum cholesterol and risk of Alzheimer disease: a community-based cohort study. *Neurology,* 2005, 65, 1045-1050.

Lindberg, G; Larsson, G; Setterlind, S; Råstam, L. Serum lipids and mood in working men and women in Sweden. *Epidemiol Community Health,* 1994, 48, 360–363.

Lindberg, G; Råstam, L; Gullberg, B; Eklund, GA. Low serum cholesterol concentration and short term mortality from injuries in men and women. *BMJ,* 1992, 305, 277-279.

Lowry, OH; Rosenbrough, NJ; Farr, AL; Randall, RJ. Protein measurement with the Folin phenol reagent. *J Biol Chem,* 1951, 193, 265-275.

Maes, M; Delanghe, J; Meltzer, HY; Scharpé, S; D'Hondt, P; Cosyns, P. Lower degree of esterification of serum cholesterol in depression: Relevance for depression and suicide research. *Acta Psychiatr Scand,* 1994, 90, 252– 258.

Maes, M; Smith, R; Christophe, A; Vandoolaeghe, E; Van Gastel, A; Neels, H; Demedts, P; Wauters, A; Meltzer, HY. Lower serum high-density lipoprotein cholesterol (HDL-C) in major depression and in depressed men with serious suicidal attempts: Relationship with immune inflammatory markers. *Acta Psychiatr Scand,* 1997, 95, 212–221.

Malone, KM; Thase, ME; Mieczkowski, T; Myers, JE; Stull, SD; Cooper, TB; Mann, JJ. Fenfluramine challenge test as a predictor of outcome in major depression. *Psychopharmacol Bull,* 1993, 29, 155-161.

Marazziti, D; Lenzi, A; Galli, L; San Martino, S; Cassano, GB. Decreased platelet serotonin uptake in bipolar I patients. *Int Clin Psychopharmacol,* 1991, 6, 25-30.

Marcinko, D; Bilic, V; Pivac, N; Tentor, B; Franic, T; Loncar, M; Marcinko, VM; Jakovljevic, M. Serum cholesterol concentration and structured individual psychoanalytic psychotherapy insuicidal and non-suicidal male patients suffering from borderline personality disorder. *Coll Antropol,* 2011, 35, (Suppl 1), 219-223.

Marcinko, D; Martinac, M; Karlovic, D; Loncar, C. Cholesterol serum levels in violent and non-violent young male schizophrenic suicide attempters. *Psychiatr Danub,* 2004, 16, 161-164.

Marcinko, D; Martinac, M; Karlovic, D; Filipcic, I; Loncar, C; Pivac, N; Jakovljevic, M. Are there differences in serum cholesterol and cortisol concentrations between violent and non-violent schizophrenic male suicide attempters? *Coll Antropol,* 2005, 29, 153-157.

Marcinko, D; Pivac, N; Martinac, M; Jakovljevic, M; Mihaljevic-Peles, A; Muck-Seler D. Platelet serotonin and serum cholesterol concentrations in suicidal and non-suicidal male patients with a first episode of psychosis. *Psychiatry Res,* 2007, 150, 105-108.

Mauch, DH; Nägler, K; Schumacher, S; Göritz, C; Müller, EC; Otto, A; Pfrieger, FW. CNS synaptogenesis promoted by glia-derived cholesterol. *Science,* 2001, 294, 1354-1357.

Maxfield, FR; Tabas, I. Role of cholesterol and lipid organization in disease. *Nature,* 2005, 438, 612-621.

McCallum, J; Simons, L; Simons, J; Friedlander, Y. Low serum cholesterol is not associated with depression in the elderly: Data from an Australian community study. *Aust N Z J Med,* 1994, 24, 561– 564.

McKhann, G; Drachman, D; Folstein, M; Katzman, R; Price, D; Stadlan, EM. Clinical diagnosis of Alzheimer's disease: report of the NINCDS-ADRDA Work Group under the auspices of Department of Health and Human

Services Task Force on Alzheimer's Disease. *Neurology,* 1984, 34, 939-944.

McMahon, FJ; Buervenich, S; Charney, D; Lipsky, R; Rush, AJ; Wilson, AF; Sorant, AJ; Papanicolaou, GJ; Laje, G; Fava, M; Trivedi, MH; Wisniewski, SR; Manji, H. Variation in the gene encoding the serotonin 2A receptor is associated with outcome of antidepressant treatment. *Am J Hum Genet,* 2006, 78, 804-814.

McPherson, S; Back, C; Buckwalter, JG; Cummings, JL. Gender-related cognitive deficits in Alzheimer's disease. *Int Psychogeriatr,* 1999, 11, 117-122.

Meagher, JB; O'Halloran, A; Carney, PA; Leonard, BE. Changes in platelet 5-hydroxytryptamine uptake in mania. *J Affect Disord,* 1990, 19, 191-196.

Meltzer, HY; Maes, M. Pindolol pretreatment blocks stimulation by meta-chlorophenylpiperazine of prolactin but not cortisol secretion in normal men. *Psychiatry Res,* 1995, 58, 89-98.

Merched, A; Xia, Y; Visvikis, S; Serot, JM; Siest, G. Decreased high-density lipoprotein cholesterol and serum apolipoprotein AI concentrations are highly correlated with the severity of Alzheimer's disease. *Neurobiol Aging,* 2000, 21, 27-30.

Meszaros, Z; Borcsiczky, D; Mate, M; Tarcali, J; Tekes, K, Magyar, K. MAO inhibitory side effects of neuroleptics and platelet serotonin content in schizophrenic patients. *J Neural Transm Suppl,* 1998, 52, 79-85.

Meyer, JM; Koro, CE. The effects of antipsychotic therapy on serum lipids: a comprehensive review. *Schizophr Res,* 2004, 70, 1-17.

Michikawa, M. Cholesterol paradox: is high total or low HDL cholesterol level a risk for Alzheimer's disease? *J Neurosci Res,* 2003, 72, 141-146.

Michikawa, M; Yanagisawa, K. Inhibition of cholesterol production but not of nonsterol isoprenoid products induces neuronal cell death. *J Neurochem,* 1999, 72, 2278-2285.

Mielke, MM; Zandi, PP; Sjögren, M; Gustafson, D; Ostling, S; Steen, B; Skoog, I. High total cholesterol levels in late life associated with a reduced risk of dementia. *Neurology,* 2005, 64, 1689-1695.

Miller, KJ. Serotonin 5-ht2c receptor agonists: potential for the treatment of obesity. *Mol Interv,* 2005, 5, 282-291.

Modai, I; Valevski, A; Dror, S; Weizman, A. Serum cholesterol levels and suicidal tendencies in psychiatric inpatients. *J Clin Psychiatry,* 1994, 55, 252-254.

Modai, I; Zemishlany, Z; Jerushalmy, Z. 5-hydroxytryptamine uptake by blood platelets of unipolar and bipolar depressed patients. *Neuropsychobiology,* 1984, 12, 93-95

Morgan, RE; Palinkas, LA; Barrett-Connor, EL; Wingard, DL. Plasma cholesterol and depressive symptoms in older men. *Lancet,* 1993, 341, 75–79.

Muck-Seler, D; Jakovljevic, M; Deanovic, Z. Platelet serotonin in subtypes of schizophrenia and unipolar depression. *Psychiatry Res,* 1991, 38, 105-113.

Muck-Seler, D; Jakovljevic, M; Pivac, N. Platelet 5-HT concentrations and suicidal behavior in recurrent major depression. *J Affect Disord,* 1996, 39, 73–80.

Muck-Seler, D; Sagud, M; Mihaljevic-Peles, A; Jakovljevic, M; Pivac, N. Baseline lipid levels and acute treatment response to paroxetine and tianeptine in depressed women. *J Clin Psychopharmacol,* 2011, 31, 387-390.

Mulder, M; Ravid, R; Swaab, DF; de Kloet, ER; Haasdijk, ED; Julk, J; van der Boom, JJ; Havekes, LM. Reduced levels of cholesterol, phospholipids, and fatty acids in cerebrospinal fluid of Alzheimer disease patients are not related to apolipoprotein E4. *Alzheimer Dis Assoc Disord,* 1998, 12, 198-203.

Muldoon, MF; Kaplan, JR; Manuck, SB; Mann, JJ. Effects of a low-fat diet on brain serotonergic responsivity in cynomolgus monkeys. *Biol Psychiatry,* 1992, 31, 739-742.

Muldoon, MF; Mackey, RH; Korytkowski, MT; Flory, JD; Pollock, BG, Manuck, SB. The metabolic syndrome is associated with reduced central serotonergic responsivity in healthy community volunteers. *J Clin Endocrinol Metab,* 2006, 91, 718-721.

Muldoon, MF; Manuck, SB; Matthews, KA. Lowering cholesterol concentrations and mortality: a quantitative review of primary prevention trials. *BMJ,* 1990, 301, 309-314.

Muldoon, MF; Manuck, SB; Mendelsohn, AB; Kaplan, JR; Belle, SH. Cholesterol reduction and non-illness mortality: meta-analysis of randomised clinical trials. *BMJ,* 2001, 322, 11-15.

Muller-Oerlinghausen, B; Roggenbach, J; Franke, L. Serotonergic platelet markers of suicidal behavior--do they really exist? *J Affect Disord,* 2004, 79, 13-24.

Nacmias, B; Tedde, A; Forleo, P; Piacentini, S; Guarnieri, BM; Bartoli, A; Ortenzi, L; Petruzzi, C, Serio, A; Marcon, G, Sorbi, S. Association between 5-HT(2A) receptor polymorphism and psychotic symptoms in Alzheimer's disease. *Biol Psychiatry,* 2001, 50, 472-475.

Nakamura, T; Matsushita, S; Nishiguchi, N, Kimura, M, Yoshino, A, Higuchi, S. Association of a polymorphism of the 5HT2A receptor gene promoter region with alcohol dependence. *Mol Psychiatry,* 1999, 4, 85-88.

Nakao, M; Yamanaka, G; Kuboki, T. Major depression and somatic symptoms in a mind/body medicine clinic. *Psychopathology,* 2001, 34, 230-235.

Nakao, M; Yano, E. Relationship between major depression and high serum cholesterol in Japanese men. *Tohoku J Exp Med,* 2004, 204, 273-287.

Neaton, JD; Blackburn, H; Jacobs, D; Kuller, L; Lee, DJ; Sherwin, R, Shih, J; Stamler, J; Wentworth, D. Serum cholesterol level and mortality findings for men screened in the Multiple Risk Factor Intervention Trial. Multiple Risk Factor Intervention Trial Research Group. *Arch Intern Med,* 1992, 152, 1490-1500.

Nonogaki, K; Strack, AM; Dallman, MF, Tecott, LH. Leptin-independent hyperphagia and type 2 diabetes in mice with a mutated serotonin 5-HT2C receptor gene. *Nat Med,* 1998, 4, 1152-1156.

Norata, GD; Pirillo, A; Catapano, AL. Modified HDL: biological and physiopathological consequences. *Nutr Metab Cardiovasc Dis,* 2006, 16, 371-386.

Notkola, IL; Sulkava, R; Pekkanen, J; Erkinjuntti, T; Ehnholm, C; Kivinen, P; Tuomilehto, J; Nissinen, A. Serum total cholesterol, apolipoprotein E epsilon 4 allele, and Alzheimer's disease. *Neuroepidemiology,* 1998, 17, 14-20.

O'Driscoll, G; Green, D; Taylor, RR. Simvastatin, an HMG-coenzyme A reductase inhibitor, improves endothelial function within 1 month. *Circulation,* 1997, 95, 1126-1131.

Olajossy-Hilkesberger, L; Godlewska, B; Marmurowska-Michałowskal, H; Olajossy, M; Landowski, J. Antipsychotic-induced weight gain--pharmacogenetic studies. *Psychiatr Pol,* 2006, 40, 1009-1020.

Olusi, SO; Fido, AA. Serum lipid concentrations in patients with major depressive disorder. *Biol Psychiatry,* 1996, 40, 1128–1131.

Ormiston, T; Wolkowitz, OM; Reus, VI; Manfredi, F. Behavioral implications of lowering cholesterol levels: a double-blind pilot study. *Psychosomatics,* 2003, 44, 412-414

Overall, JE; Gorham, DR. The Brief Psychiatric Rating Scale. *Psychological Research,* 1962, 10, 799–812.

Oxenkrug, GF. The content and uptake of 5-HT by blood platelets in depressive patients. *J Neural Transm,* 1979, 45, 285-289.

Oxenkrug, GF; Branconnier, RJ; Harto-Traux, N; Cole, JO. Is serum cholesterol a biological marker for major depressive episode? *Am J Psychiatry,* 1983, 140, 920–921.

Pae, CU; Kim, JJ, Lee, SJ; Lee, C; Paik, IH; Lee, CU. Aberration of cholesterol level in first-onset bipolar I patients. *J Affect Disord,* 2004, 83, 79-82.

Panza, F; D'Introno, A; Colacicco, AM, Capurso, C; Pichichero, G; Capurso, SA; Capurso, A; Solfrizzi, V. Lipid metabolism in cognitive decline and dementia. *Brain Res Rev,* 2006, 51, 275–292.

Papakostas, GI; Iosifescu, DV; Petersen, T; Hamill, SK; Alpert, JE; Nierenberg, AA; Rosenbaum, JF; Fava, M. Serum cholesterol in the continuation phase of pharmacotherapy with fluoxetine in remitted major depressive disorder. *J Clin Psychopharmacol,* 2004a, 24, 467-469.

Papakostas, GI; Ongür, D; Iosifescu, DV; Mischoulon, D; Fava, M. Cholesterol in mood and anxiety disorders: review of the literature and new hypotheses. *Eur Neuropsychopharmacol,* 2004b, 14, 135-142.

Papakostas, GI; Petersen, T; Mischoulon, D; Hughes, ME; Alpert, JE; Nierenberg, AA; Rosenbaum, JF; Fava, M. Serum cholesterol and serotonergic function in major depressive disorder. *Psychiatry Res,* 2003a, 118, 137-145.

Papakostas, GI; Petersen, T; Sonawalla, SB; Merens, W; Iosifescu, DV; Alpert, JE; Fava, M; Nierenberg, AA. Serum cholesterol in treatment-resistant depression. *Neuropsychobiology,* 2003b, 47,146-151.

Papassotiropoulos, A; Hawellek, B; Frahnert, C; Rao, GS, Rao, ML. The risk of acute suicidality in psychiatric inpatients increases with low plasma cholesterol. *Pharmacopsychiatry,* 1999, 32, 1-4.

Partonen, T; Haukka, J, Virtamo, J; Taylor, PR; Lönnqvist, J. Association of low serum total cholesterol with major depression and suicide. *Br J Psychiatry,* 1999, 175, 259-262.

Penttinen, J. Hypothesis: low serum cholesterol, suicide, and interleukin-2. *Am J Epidemiol,* 1995, 141, 716-718.

Perez-Rodriguez, MM; Baca-Garcia, E , Diaz-Sastre, C , Garcia-Resa, E , Ceverino, A; Saiz-Ruiz, J; Oquendo, MA; de Leon, J. Low serum cholesterol may be associated with suicide attempt history. *J Clin Psychiatry,* 2008, 69, 1920-1927.

Perticone, F; Ceravolo, R; Maio, R; Cloro, C; Candigliota, M; Scozzafava, A; Mongiardo, A; Mastroroberto, P; Chello, M; Mattioli, PL. Effects of atorvastatin and vitamin C on endothelial function of hypercholesterolemic patients. *Atherosclerosis,* 2000, 152, 511-518.

Peter, H; Hand, I; Hohagen, F; Koenig, A; Mindermann, O; Oeder, F; Wittich, M. Serum cholesterol level comparison: control subjects, anxiety disorder patients, and obsessive-compulsive disorder patients. *Can J Psychiatry,* 2002, 47, 557-561.

Pfrieger, FW. Cholesterol homeostasis and function in neurons of the central nervous system. *Cell Mol Life Sci,* 2003, 60, 1158-1171.

Pivac, N; Jakovljevic, M; Muck-Seler, D; Brzovic, Z. Hypothalamic–pituitary–adrenal axis function and platelet serotonin concentrations in depressed patients. *Psychiatry Research,* 1997, 73, 123–132.

Pivac, N; Knezevic, J; Mustapic, M; Dezeljin, M; Muck-Seler, D; Kozaric-Kovacic, D, Balija, M; Matijevic, T; Pavelic, J. The lack of association between monoamine oxidase (MAO) intron 13 polymorphism and platelet MAO-B activity among men. *Life Sci,* 2006a, 79, 45-49.

Pivac, N; Kozaric-Kovacic, D; Mustapic, M; Dezeljin, M; Borovecki, A; Grubisic-Ilic, M; Muck-Seler, D. Platelet serotonin in combat related posttraumatic stress disorder with psychotic symptoms. *J Affect Disord,* 2006b, 93, 223-227.

Pivac, N; Muck-Seler, D; Barisic, I; Jakovljevic, M; Puretic, Z. Platelet serotonin concentration in dialysis patients with somatic symptoms of depression. *Life Sci,* 2001, 68, 2423-2433.

Pivac, N; Muck-Seler, D; Mustapic, M; Nenadic-Sviglin, K; Kozaric-Kovacic, D. Platelet serotonin concentration in alcoholic subjects. *Life Sci,* 2004, 76, 521-531.

Pjrek, E; Winkler, D; Abramson, DW; Konstantinidis, A; Stastny, J; Willeit, M; Praschak-Rieder, N; Kasper, S. Serum lipid levels in seasonal affective disorder. *Eur Arch Psychiatry Clin Neurosci,* 2007, 257, 197-202.

Polk, DM; Naqvi, TZ. Cardiovascular disease in women: sex differences in presentation, risk factors, and evaluation. *Curr Cardiol Rep,* 2005, 7, 166-172.

Pozzi, F; Troisi, A; Cerilli, M; Autore, AM; Lo Castro, C; Ribatti, D; Frajese, G. Serum cholesterol and impulsivity in a large sample of healthy young men. *Psychiatry Res,* 2003, 120, 239-245.

Presecki, P; Muck-Seler, D, Mimica, N, Pivac, N; Mustapic, M; Stipcevic, T; Smalc, VF. Serum lipid levels in patients with Alzheimer's disease. *Coll Antropol,* 2011, 35, Suppl 1, 115-120.

Pucadyil, TJ; Chattopadhyay, A. Cholesterol depletion induces dynamic confinement of the G-protein coupled serotonin(1A) receptor in the plasma membrane of living cells. *Biochim Biophys Acta,* 2007, 1768, 655-668.

Puglielli, L. Aging of the brain, neurotrophin signaling, and Alzheimer's disease: is IGF1-R the common culprit? *Neurobiol Aging,* 2008, 29, 795-811.

Rabe-Jablonska, J; Poprawska, I. Levels of serum total cholesterol and LDL-cholesterol in patients with major depression in acute period and remission. *Med Sci Monit,* 2000, 6, 539–547.

Raeder, MB; Bjelland, I; Emil Vollset, S; Steen, VM. Obesity, dyslipidemia, and diabetes with selective serotonin reuptake inhibitors: the Hordaland Health Study. *J Clin Psychiatry,* 2006, 67, 1974-1982.

Rafter, D. Biochemical markers of anxiety and depression. *Psychiatry Res,* 2001, 103, 93–96.

Ramdane, S; Daoudi-Gueddah, D. Mild hypercholesterolemia, normal plasma triglycerides, and normal glucose levels across dementia staging in Alzheimer's disease: a clinical setting-based retrospective study. *Am J Alzheimers Dis Other Demen,* 2011, 26, 399-405.

Refolo, LM; Pappolla, MA; LaFrancois, J; Malester, B; Schmidt, SD; Thomas-Bryant, T; Tint, GS; Wang, R; Mercken, M; Petanceska, SS; Duff, KE. A cholesterol-lowering drug reduces beta-amyloid pathology in a transgenic mouse model of Alzheimer's disease. *Neurobiol Dis*, 2001, 8, 890-899.

Regitz-Zagrosek, V; Lehmkuhl, E; Mahmoodzadeh, S. Gender aspects of the role of the metabolic syndrome as a risk factor for cardiovascular disease. *Gend Med,* 2007, 4, Suppl B, 162-177.

Reitz, C; Tang, MX; Luchsinger, J; Mayeux, R. Relation of plasma lipids to Alzheimer disease and vascular dementia. *Arch Neurol,* 2004, 61, 705-714.

Reitz, C; Tang, MX; Schupf, N; Manly, JJ; Mayeux, R; Luchsinger, JA. Association of higher levels of high-density lipoprotein cholesterol in elderly individuals and lower risk of late-onset Alzheimer disease. *Arch Neurol,* 2010, 67, 1491-1497.

Richards, JC; Hof, A; Alvarenga, M. Serum lipids and their relationships with hostility and angry affect and behaviors in men. *Health Psychol,* 2000, 19, 393-398.

Ringo, DL; Lindley, SE; Faull, KF; Faustman, WO. Cholesterol and serotonin: seeking a possible link between blood cholesterol and CSF 5-HIAA. *Biol Psychiatry,* 1994, 35, 957-959.

Rosmond, R; Bouchard, C; Björntorp, P. 5-HT2A receptor gene promoter polymorphism in relation to abdominal obesity and cortisol. *Obes Res,* 2002, 10, 585-589.

Rothe, C; Koszycki, D, Bradwejn, J; King, N; De Luca, V; Shaikh, S; Franke, P; Garritsen, H; Fritze, J; Deckert, J; Kennedy, JL. Association study of serotonin-2A receptor gene polymorphism and panic disorder in patients from Canada and Germany. *Neurosci Lett,* 2004, 363, 276-279.

Saari, K; Koponen, H; Laitinen, J; Jokelainen, J; Lauren, L; Isohanni, M; Lindeman, S; Hyperlipidemia in persons using antipsychotic medication: a general population-based birth cohort study. *J Clin Psychiatry,* 2004, 65, 547-550.

Sagud, M; Mihaljevic-Peles, A; Pivac, N; Jakovljevic, M; Muck-Seler, D. Platelet serotonin and lipid levels in psychotic mania. *J Affect Disord,* 2007, 9, 247-251.

Sagud, M; Mihaljevic-Peles, A; Pivac, N; Jakovljevic, M; Muck-Seler, D. Lipid levels in female patients with affective disorders. *Psychiatry Res,* 2009, 168, 218-221.

Sampietro, T; Bigazzi, F; Dal Pino, B, Puntoni, M, Bionda, A. HDL: the 'new' target of cardiovascular medicine. *Int J Cardiol,* 2006, 108, 143-154.

Sarchiapone, M; Camardese, G; Roy, AC; Della Casa, S; Satta, MA; Gonzalez, B; Berman, J; De Risio, S. Cholesterol and serotonin indices in depressed and suicidal patients. *J Affect Disord*, 2001, 62, 217–219.

Sarchiapone, M; Roy, A, Camardese, G; De Risio, S. Further evidence for low serum cholesterol and suicidal behaviour. *J Affect Disord,* 2000, 61, 69-71.

Saxena, R; Sitholey, P; Saxena, AK; Vrat, S; Kumar, S; Shanker, K. Platelet serotonin in juvenile mania. *Biogenic Amines*, 1999, 15, 413–421.

Scanlon, SM; Williams, DC; Schloss, P. Membrane cholesterol modulates serotonin transporter activity. *Biochemistry,* 2001, 40, 10507-10513.

Schreiber, R; De Vry, J. Role of 5-hT2C receptors in the hypophagic effect of m-CPP, ORG 37684 and CP-94,253 in the rat. Prog Neuropsychopharmacol *Biol Psychiatry,* 2002, 26, 441-449.

Schneider, LS; Dagerman, KS. Psychosis of Alzheimer's disease: clinical characteristics and history. *J Psychiatr Res,* 2004, 38, 105-111.

Seneviratne, SL; Warnasooriya, WM; Gunatilake, SB; Fonseka, MM, Gunawardena, MK; de Silva, HJ. Serum cholesterol concentrations in parasuicide. *Ceylon Med J,* 1999, 44, 11-13.

Serretti, A; Calati, R; Mandelli, L; De Ronchi, D. Serotonin transporter gene variants and behavior: a comprehensive review. *Curr Drug Targets,* 2006, 7, 1659-1669.

Sevincok, L; Buyukozturk, A; Dereboy, F. Serum lipid concentrations in patients with comorbid generalized anxiety disorder and major depressive disorder. *Can J Psychiatry,* 2001, 46, 68-71.

Shea, MT; Pilkonis, PA; Beckham, E; Collins, JF; Elkin, I; Sotsky, SM; Docherty, JP. Personality disorders and treatment outcome in the NIMH Treatment of Depression Collaborative Research Program. *Am J Psychiatry,* 1990, 147, 711-718.

Shibata, H; Kumagai, S; Watanabe, S; Suzuki, T. Relationship of serum cholesterols and vitamin E to depressive status in the elderly. *J Epidemiol,* 1999, 9, 261-267.

Shie, FS; Jin, LW; Cook, DG; Leverenz, JB; LeBoeuf, RC. Diet-induced hypercholesterolemia enhances brain A beta accumulation in transgenic mice. *Neuroreport,* 2002, 13, 455-459.

Shimokawa, H; Vanhoutte, PM. Impaired endothelium-dependent relaxation to aggregating platelets and related vasoactive substances in porcine coronary arteries in hypercholesterolemia and atherosclerosis. *Circ Res,* 1989, 64, 900-914.

Shively, CA; Register, TC; Friedman, DP; Morgan, TM; Thompson, J; Lanier, T. Social stress-associated depression in adult female cynomolgus monkeys (Macaca fascicularis). *Biol Psychol,* 2005, 69, 67-84.

Shobab, LA; Hsiung, GY; Feldman, HH. Cholesterol in Alzheimer's disease. *Lancet Neurol,* 2005, 4, 841-852.

Singh-Manoux, A; Gimeno, D; Kivimaki, M, Brunner, E, Marmot, MG. Low HDL cholesterol is a risk factor for deficit and decline in memory in midlife: the Whitehall II study. *Arterioscler Thromb Vasc Biol,* 2008, 28, 1556-1562.

Smith, CC; Betteridge, DJ. Reduced platelet serotonin content and release in familial hypercholesterolaemia. *Atherosclerosis,* 1997, 130, 87-92.

Smoller, JW; Biederman, J; Arbeitman, L; Doyle, AE; Fagerness, J; Perlis, RH; Sklar, P; Faraone, SV. Association between the 5HT1B receptor gene (HTR1B) and the inattentive subtype of ADHD. *Biol Psychiatry,* 2006, 59, 460-467.

Sobczak, S; Honig, A; Christophe, A; Maes, M; Helsdingen, RW, De Vriese, SA; Riedel, WJ. Lower high-density lipoprotein cholesterol and increased omega-6 polyunsaturated fatty acids in first-degree relatives of bipolar patients. *Psychol Med,* 2004, 34, 103-112.

Solfrizzi, V; D'Introno, A; Colacicco, AM; Capurso, C; Todarello, O; Pellicani, V; Capurso, SA; Pietrarossa, G; Santamato, V; Capurso, A; Panza, F. Circulating biomarkers of cognitive decline and dementia. *Clin Chim Acta,* 2006, 364, 91-112.

Solomon, A; Leoni, V; Kivipelto, M; Besga, A; Oksengård, AR; Julin, P; Svensson, L; Wahlund, LO; Andreasen, N; Winblad, B; Soininen, H; Björkhem, I. Plasma levels of 24S-hydroxycholesterol reflect brain volumes in patients without objective cognitive impairment but not in those with Alzheimer's disease. *Neurosci Lett,* 2009, 462, 89-93.

Sonawalla, SB; Papakostas, GI; Petersen, TJ; Yeung, AS; Smith, MM; Sickinger, AH; Gordon, J; Israel, JA; Tedlow, JR; Lamon-Fava, S; Fava, M. Elevated cholesterol levels associated with nonresponse to fluoxetine treatment in major depressive disorder. *Psychosomatics,* 2002, 43, 310-316.

Song, F; Poljak, A; Smythe, GA; Sachdev, P. Plasma biomarkers for mild cognitive impairment and Alzheimer's disease. *Brain Res Rev,* 2009, 61, 69-80.

Sooksawate, T; Simmonds, MA. Increased membrane cholesterol reduces the potentiation of GABA(A) currents by neurosteroids in dissociated hippocampal neurones. *Neuropharmacology,* 1998, 37, 1103-1110.

Sooksawate, T; Simmonds, MA. Effects of membrane cholesterol on the sensitivity of the GABA(A) receptor to GABA in acutely dissociated rat hippocampal neurones. *Neuropharmacology,* 2001, 40, 178-184.

Stahl, SM; Woo, DJ, Mefford, IN; Berger, PA; Ciaranello, RD. Hyperserotonemia and platelet serotonin uptake and release in schizophrenia and affective disorders. *Am J Psychiatry,* 1983, 140, 26-30.

Steegmans, PH; Fekkes, D; Hoes, AW; Bak, AA; van der Does, E; Grobbee, DE. Low serum cholesterol concentration and serotonin metabolism in men. *BMJ,* 1996, 312, 221

Steegmans, PH; Hoes, AW; Bak, AA; van der Does, E; Grobbee, DE. Higher prevalence of depressive symptoms in middle-aged men with low serum cholesterol levels. *Psychosom Med,* 2000, 62, 205–211.

Stroes, E; de Bruin, T; de Valk, H; Erkelens, W; Banga, JD; van Rijn, H; Koomans, H; Rabelink, T. NO activity in familial combined hyperlipidemia: potential role of cholesterol remnants. *Cardiovasc Res,* 1997, 36, 445-452.

Stroes, ES; Koomans, HA; de Bruin, TW; Rabelink, TJ. Vascular function in the forearm of hypercholesterolaemic patients off and on lipid-lowering medication. *Lancet,* 1995, 346, 467-471.

Suarez, EC. Relations of trait depression and anxiety to low lipid and lipoprotein concentrations in healthy young adult women. *Psychosom Med,* 1999, 61, 273–279.

Sudhop, T; Bauer, J, Elger, CE; von Bergmann, K. Increased high-density lipoprotein cholesterol in patients with epilepsy treated with carbamazepine: a gender-related study. *Epilepsia,* 1999, 40, 480-484.

Sullivan, PF; Joyce, PR; Bulik, CM; Mulder, RT; Oakley-Browne, M. Total cholesterol and suicidality in depression. *Biol Psychiatry,* 1994, 36, 472-477.

Suzuki, M; Wright, LS; Marwah, P; Lardy, HA; Svendsen, CN. Mitotic and neurogenic effects of dehydroepiandrosterone (DHEA) on human neural stem cell cultures derived from the fetal cortex. *Proc Natl Acad Sci USA,* 2004, 101, 3202–3207.

Svenningsson, P; Chergui, K; Rachleff, I; Flajolet, M; Zhang, X; El Yacoubi, M, Vaugeois, JM; Nomikos, GG; Greengard, P. Alterations in 5-HT1B receptor function by p11 in depression-like states. *Science,* 2006, 311, 77-80.

Taïeb, N; Yahi, N; Fantini, J. Rafts and related glycosphingolipid-enriched microdomains in the intestinal epithelium: bacterial targets linked to nutrient absorption. *Adv Drug Deliv Rev,* 2004; 56, 779–794.

Takahashi, S. Reduction of blood platelet serotonin levels in manic and depressed patients. *Folia Psychiatr Neurol Jpn,* 1976, 30, 475-486.

Takahashi, S. Monoamine oxidase activity in blood platelets from manic and depressed patients. *Folia Psychiatr Neurol Jpn,* 1977, 31, 37-48.

Tan, ZS; Seshadri, S; Beiser, A; Wilson, PW; Kiel, DP; Tocco, M; D'Agostino, RB; Wolf, PA. Plasma total cholesterol level as a risk factor for Alzheimer disease: the Framingham Study. *Arch Intern Med,* 2003,163, 1053-1057.

Tecott, LH; Sun, LM, Akana, SF; Strack, AM; Lowenstein, DH; Dallman, MF; Julius, D. Eating disorder and epilepsy in mice lacking 5-HT2c serotonin receptors. *Nature,* 1995, 374, 542-546.

Thelen, KM; Falkai, P; Bayer, TA; Lütjohann, D. Cholesterol synthesis rate in human hippocampus declines with aging. *Neurosci Lett,* 2006, 403, 15-19.

Terao, T; Iwata, N; Kanazawa, K; Takano, T; Takahashi, N; Hayashi, T; Sugawara, Y. Low serum cholesterol levels and depressive state in human dock visitors. *Acta Psychiatr Scand,* 2000a, 101, 231–234.

Terao, T; Nakamura, J; Yoshimura, R; Ohmori, O; Takahashi, N; Kojima, H; Soeda, S; Shinkai, T; Nakano, H; Okuno, T. Relationship between serum cholesterol levels and meta-chlorophenylpiperazine-induced cortisol responses in healthy men and women. *Psychiatry Res,* 2000b, 96, 167-173.

Terao, T; Yoshimura, R; Ohmori, O; Takano, T; Takahashi, N; Iwata, N; Suzuki, T; Abe, K. Effect of serum cholesterol levels on meta-chlorophenylpiperazine-evoked neuroendocrine responses in healthy subjects. *Biol Psychiatry,* 1997, 41, 974-978.

Thomas, AJ; Ferrier, IN; Kalaria, RN; Perry, RH; Brown, A; O'Brien, JT. A neuropathological study of vascular factors in late-life depression. *J Neurol Neurosurg Psychiatry,* 2001, 70, 83-87.

Troisi, A; D'Argenio, A. Apolipoprotein A-I/apolipoprotein B ratio and aggression in violent and nonviolent young adult males. *J Psychiatr Res,* 2006, 40, 466-472.

Troisi, A, Scucchi, S; San Martino, L; Montera, P; d'Amore, A; Moles, A. Age specificity of the relationship between serum cholesterol and mood in obese women. *Physiol Behav,* 2001, 72, 409-413.

Van Praag, HM. Functionalizing diagnostics. *Am J Psychiatry*, 2004, 161, 2138.

Verkes, RJ; Van der Mast, RC; Kerkhof, AJ; Fekkes, D; Hengeveld, MW; Tuyl, JP, Van Kempen, GM. Platelet serotonin, monoamine oxidase activity, and [3H]paroxetine binding related to impulsive suicide attempts and borderline personality disorder. *Biol Psychiatry,* 1998, 43, 740-746.

Vevera, J; Fisar, Z; Kvasnicka, T; Zdenek, H; Stárková, L; Ceska, R; Papezová, H. Cholesterol-lowering therapy evokes time-limited changes in serotonergic transmission. *Psychiatry Res,* 2005, 133, 197-203.

Vevera, J; Zukov, I; Morcinek, T; Papezová, H. Cholesterol concentrations in violent and non-violent women suicide attempters. *Eur Psychiatry,* 2003, 18, 23-27.

Videtic, A; Pungercic, G; Pajnic, IZ; Zupanc, T; Balazic, J; Tomori, M; Komel, R. Association study of seven polymorphisms in four serotonin receptor genes on suicide victims. *Am J Med Genet B Neuropsychiatr Genet,* 2006, 141B, 669-672.

Villacres, EC; Hollifield, M; Katon, WJ; Wilkinson, CW; Veith, RC. Sympathetic nervous system activity in panic disorder. *Psychiatry Res,* 1987, 21, 313-321.

Vimaleswaran, KS; Zhao, JH; Wainwright, NW; Surtees, PG; Wareham, NJ; Loos, RJ. Association between serotonin 5-HT-2C receptor gene (HTR2C) polymorphisms and obesity- and mental health-related phenotypes in a large population-based cohort. *Int J Obes* (Lond), 2010, 34, 1028-1033.

Virkkunen, M. Serum cholesterol levels in homicidal offenders. A low cholesterol level is connected with a habitually violent tendency under the influence of alcohol. *Neuropsychobiology,* 1983, 10, 65-69.

Wahrle, S; Das, P; Nyborg, AC; McLendon, C; Shoji, M; Kawarabayashi, T; Younkin, LH; Younkin, SG; Golde, TE. Cholesterol-dependent gamma-secretase activity in buoyant cholesterol-rich membrane microdomains. *Neurobiol Dis,* 2002, 9, 11-23.

Wallner, B; Machatschke, IH. The evolution of violence in men: the function of central cholesterol and serotonin. *Prog Neuropsychopharmacol Biol Psychiatry,* 2009, 33, 391-397.

Wang, JM; Irwin, RW; Liu, L; Chen, S; Brinton, RD. Regeneration in a degenerating brain: potential of allopregnanolone as a neuroregenerative agent. *Curr Alzheimer Res,* 2007, 4, 510-517.

Wang, JM; Johnston, PB; Ball, BG; Brinton, RD. The neurosteroid allopregnanolone promotes proliferation of rodent and human neural progenitor cells and regulates cell-cycle gene and protein expression. *J Neurosci,* 2005, 25, 4706–4718.

Weidner, G; Connor, SL; Hollis, JF, Connor, WE. Improvements in hostility and depression in relation to dietary change and cholesterol lowering: The Family Heart Study. *Ann Intern Med,* 1992, 117, 820– 823.

Weisler, RH; Keck, PE Jr; Swann, AC; Cutler, AJ; Ketter, TA, Kalali, AH. SPD417 Study Group. Extended-release carbamazepine capsules as monotherapy for acute mania in bipolar disorder: a multicenter, randomized, double-blind, placebo-controlled trial. *J Clin Psychiatry,* 2005, 66, 323-330.

Whitfield, JF. Can statins put the brakes on Alzheimer's disease? *Expert Opin Investig Drugs,* 2006, 15, 1479-1485.

Williams, TI; Lynn, BC; Markesbery, WR; Lovell, MA. Increased levels of 4-hydroxynonenal and acrolein, neurotoxic markers of lipid peroxidation, in the brain in Mild Cognitive Impairment and early Alzheimer's disease. *Neurobiol Aging,* 2006, 27, 1094-1099.

Williams, J; McGuffin, P; Nöthen, M; Owen, MJ. Meta-analysis of association between the 5-HT2a receptor T102C polymorphism and schizophrenia. EMASS Collaborative Group. European Multicentre Association Study of Schizophrenia. *Lancet,* 1997, 349, 1221.

Wilson, PW; D'Agostino, RB; Levy, D; Belanger, AM; Silbershatz, H; Kannel, WB. Prediction of coronary heart disease using risk factor categories. *Circulation,* 1998, 97, 1837-1847.

Wolf, H; Hensel, A, Arendt, T; Kivipelto, M; Winblad, B; Gertz, HJ. Serum lipids and hippocampal volume: the link to Alzheimer's disease? *Ann Neurol,* 2004, 56, 745-748.

Wolozin, B; Kellman, W; Ruosseau, P; Celesia, GG; Siegel, G. Decreased prevalence of Alzheimer disease associated with 3-hydroxy-3-methyglutaryl coenzyme A reductase inhibitors. *Arch Neurol,* 2000, 57, 1439-1443.

World Health Organization, The ICD-10, Classification of mental and behavioral disorders, 10 revision, Geneva, *World Health Organization,* 1992.

Yamanouchi, Y; Iwata, N; Suzuki, T; Kitajima, T; Ikeda, M; Ozaki, N. Effect of DRD2, 5-HT2A, and COMT genes on antipsychotic response to risperidone. *Pharmacogenomics J,* 2003, 3, 356-361.

Yang, Y; Yan, B, Fu, M; Xu, Y; Tian, Y. Relationship between plasma lipid concentrations and HDL subclasses. *Clin Chim Acta,* 2005, 354, 49-58.

Ying, S; Liu, XM; Sun, YM; Pan, SH. Genetic polymorphism c.1438A>G of the 5-HT(2A) receptor is associated with abdominal obesity in Chinese Northern Han population. *Mol Biol Rep,* 2009, 36, 91-95.

Young, RC; Biggs, JT; Ziegler, VE; Meyer, DA. A rating scale for mania: reliability, validity and sensitivity. *Br J Psychiatry,* 1978, 133, 429-435.

Zhang, J; McKeown, RE; Hussey, JR; Thompson, SJ; Woods, JR; Ainsworth, BE. Low HDL cholesterol is associated with suicide attempt among young healthy women: the Third National Health and Nutrition Examination Survey. *J Affect Disord,* 2005, 89, 25-33.

Zureik, M; Courbon, D; Ducimetière, P. Serum cholesterol concentration and death from suicide in men: Paris prospective study I. *BMJ,* 1996, 313, 649-651.

In: Triglycerides
Editors: C. Araujo and D. Perez
ISBN: 978-1-62417-727-9

Chapter 2

THE ROLE OF CIRCADIAN CLOCKS IN ABSORPTION AND METABOLISM OF DIETARY TRIGLYCERIDE

Xiaoyue Pan*
Department of Cell Biology and Pediatrics,
SUNY Downstate Medical Center,
Brooklyn, New York, US

ABSTRACT

Hyperlipidemia is a major risk factor for cardiovascular disease. And there is evidence to suggest that plasma lipids exhibit diurnal variations. Light is known to affect diurnal variations by entraining cells in the suprachiasmatic nucleus (SCN) of the hypothalamus region of the brain. Within these cells, positive and negative transcriptional feedback loops constitute a molecular Clock in mammals. Two transcription factors, Clock and Bmal1, play critical role in determining the circadian variations. Recent studies reveal that molecular components of the Clock system are not only in the SCN but also found within the cells of peripheral tissues, such as the gastrointestinal tract and liver. Mutant Clock gene mice are obese and show hypertriglyceridemia.

Triglyceride are the chemical form in which more than 90% of dietary fat are hydrolyzed in the intestinal lumen to free fatty acids and

* Correspondence: Xiaoyue.Pan@downstate.edu.

monoacylglycerols, which are taken up and resynthesized into triglyceride in enterocytes. Triglyceride homeostasis in the body is mainly controlled by endogenous synthesis, intestinal absorption, and hepatic metabolism. Intestinal lipid absorption and metabolism is an essential physiological process that is regulated by Clock.

This Chapter describes the molecular mechanisms that co-ordinate the absorption of triglyceride from the diet and its release into the circulation by an overview of liver cellular triglyceride metabolism and intestinal absorption regulation, as well as the function of key proteins involved in these processes, with particular emphasis on the Clock's role in triglyceride homeostasis, as it is the main target of triglyceride deposition in pathological hypertriglyceridemia. Current knowledge on Clock's role in maintaining triglyceride homeostasis and how their dysregulation leads to the pathogenesis of obesity are discussed. Future work in this area will provide a clearer picture regarding the regulation of intestinal lipid absorption and liver fat metabolism by circadian Clocks.

HIGHLIGHTS

- Circadian Clock control plasma triglyceride diurnal rhythm by modulating production and catabolism pathways key proteins and gene transcription
- The insulin and bile acid pathways accounts for a large component of insulin-dependent as well as bile acid-dependent hypertriglyceridemia
- Additional pathways (AVP, GCs) show promise as mediators of central as well as peripheral tissues Clock effects
- Alternative approaches to reducing excessive triglyceride production in metabolism syndrome are needed.

1. INTRODUCTION

Over the past few decades the classification of hypertriglyceridemia has been adjusted. Hyperlipidemia is a key physiological process that becomes altered in metabolic syndrome and represents the main target of the anti hyperlipidemia effect of statin through enhance lipoprotein catabolism and reduce plasma low-density lipoprotein cholesterol (LDL-C) and apolipoprotein (Apo) B [1;2]. At same time, Statins also can inhibit hepatic output of very-low-density lipoprotein (VLDL) apoB to decrease plasma triglyceride (TG) levels. In addition, increasing doses of rosuvastin, atorvastin and simvastatine predictably results in an incremental benefit in terms of triglyceride reduction [3]

The role of plasma triglycerides as a risk factor has routinely been identified in case–control and angiographic studies, including after adjustment total cholesterol (TC), LDL-C or high-density lipoprotein Cholesterol (HDL-C) levels [4; 5]. Some evidence studies have shown that the level of triglyceride concentration may be even more predictive in women than in men [6].

Triglyceride is one of the most important energy sources for the body in general, changes in energy expenditure associated with the light-dark cycle, induce variations in the plasma triglyceride concentration that are more gradual in humans and rodents [7]. Organisms take advantage of adapting their internal physiology to the predictable daily changes in thermogenesis, due to it enables them to anticipate these changes and to prevent unnecessary disturbance of homeostasis.

In brain, the center biological Clock, located in the suprachiasmatic nucleus (SCN) of hypothalamic receives light information through the eyes and transmits this information to the rest of the body to synchronize physiology to the periphery tissue [8-10]. Here we review several studies providing evidence for center as well as periphery tissue biological Clock control of the daily variation in several aspects of triglyceride production and catabolism. We will discussion how both hormones and the autonomic nervous system can stimulate triglyceride absorption as well as metabolism by organs in the periphery, following biological Clock control of triglyceride metabolism that mostly occur through transcription regulation system.

2. The Circadian Rhythm System

2.1. Central Oscillators

Circadian rhythms have their most acute impact, for example, when we travel across multiple time zones within a single day. Generally, most of us experience profound difficulty sleeping and maintaining routine physical performance for at least a few days as our bodies acclimate to photic stimuli and other circadian entertainers in the new environment [11]. Circadian rhythm disorder also can induce acute to chronic effects.

It is well known that circadian rhythms are programmed centrally by sunlight, allowing alignment to seasonal change of day/night cycles, and peripherally tissue by food availability. As discussed above, numerous physiological processes such as wake/sleep cycles, body temperature, hormone secretion, blood pressure, metabolic pathways, etc display diurnal variations. Nevertheless, clinical dates have indicated that several conditions such as frequent jetlag, sleep restriction or rotating shift work can disrupt these circadian rhythms and cause many metabolic disorders and cardiovascular diseases. Most recently researchers reported that 10–15% of genes expressions have shown diurnal cycles in different organs such as liver, vascular and heart. Although many of the transcription factors of the Clock system also affect metabolic regulatory activities, the molecular mechanisms driving the rhythmic expression pattern of metabolic genes have been unclear until now.

In 1994, Dr. Joseph Takahashi and his colleagues first discovered the genetic basis for the mammalian circadian Clock [12] and later in 1997, his research group cloned the mammalian circadian locomotor output cycles kaput (Clock) gene [12; 13]. They identified that intact Clock genes are necessary for normal mammalian circadian function.

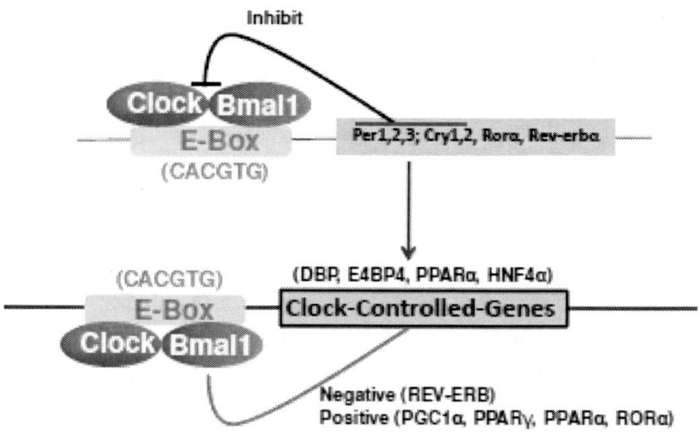

Figure 1. Clock/Bmal1 as center transcription factors to control Per/Cry as well as Clock-controlled genes. Clock and Bmal1 form heterodimers that bind to E-Box sequences to enhance the Per/Cry, Rev-erbα and ROR, Per/Cry transcription factors, move to the nucleus and repress the expression of Clock genes, constituting a negative feedback loop. In addition, Clock and Bmal1 form heterodimers and bind to E-box sequence to enhance the Clock -controlled genes such as DBP, PPARα as well HNF4α. Per/Cry also can interact with Clock-controlled genes (CCGs). CCGs can positively or negatively regulate Bmal1 gene expression.

Table 1. Circadian Clock proteins function, expression and metabolic interactions

Gene name	Func-tion	Structure	Heterdimer Bind	SCN mRNA Expression Phase Peak	SCN Protein Expression Phase Peak	Induct by Light
Clock	+	bHLH, PAS, histone acetyltransferase	Bmal1, CYC	NO	N/A	NO
Bmal1	+	bHLH, PAS	CLOCK	CT16	N/A	NO
mPer1	-	PAS,CLD	Cry1, Cry2	CT4	CT12	YES (60min)
mPer2	-	PAS,CLD	Cry1, Cry2	CT8	N/A	YES (90min)
mPer3	-	PAS,CLD,NLS	Cry1, Cry2	CT4-CT8	N/A	NO
mCry1	-	MTHF, FAD	Per1, Per2, Per3, Bmal1	CT12	CT12-CT16	NO
mCry2	-	MTHF, FAD	Per1, Per2, Per3, Bmal1	CT12	CT12-CT16	NO

NLS: Nuclear localizational signal; bHLH: basic helix-loop-helix; PAS: Per-Arnt-Sim; PHS: PAM-Highwire-RPM. CT (Circadian Time).

Following the few years, period circadian protein homolog (Per1, Per2, Per3), Cryptochromes (Cry1, Cry2), and Aryl hydrocarbon receptor nuclear translocator-like (ARNTL or Bmal1, MOP3) were cloned and their transcripts were shown to be present in the SCN of mammals. Clinical research have proposed that we can measures Per2 expression levels to tell whether a person is an early morning person or a "night owl" using a genetic test from a cheek swab [14]. Per2 has been shown to interact with Cry1 [15]. Cry1 are a class of blue light sensitive flavoproteins found in plant and animals [16].

Table 2. Selected physiological function, target genes and knock out phenotypes of molecular Clock transcription factors involving in triglyceride production and metabolism

Factor	Selected Tissue Distribution	Selected Physiology Roles	Selected Targets Genes	Phenotype of Knockout mice
Clock	Heart, hypothalamus Intestine, liver	Appetite regulation, Oleate oxidation, oxygen consumption, cell cycle regulation, lipid and glucose metabolism, Triglyceride absorption	Orexin, Ghrelin, Cart, Slc27a1, Ndufa3/b3, PPARα, Wee1, Shp, MTP, Fabp1, Acsl4, Noc	Obesity, metabolic syndrome, hyperphagia, hyperinsulinemia, hyperlipidemia, hepatic steatosis; dyregulation of ghrelin, orexin; CART, reduced arterial blood pressure, altered renal function and excretion of diluted urine (in $Clock^{-/-}$ mice)
Bmal1	Liver, adipocytes, intestine	Glucose mobilization, adipogenesis; cell cycle regulation	Slc37a4, PCK2, AK3l1, Slc2a2, PPARγ2, Ap2, Srebp1c, Srebp1α, C/EBPs, FAS, Noc	Hypoglycemia, impaired glucose clearance, reduced life span, premature aging, impaired stroidogenesis, reduced fertility; impaired adipogenesis, abolished oscillations in plasma glucose and triglycerides, fasting hypoglycemia (in liver-specific KO), Diabetes mellitus (in –pancreas-specific KO)
Per	Hypothalamus Intestine, liver	Tumor suppressor, cell cycle regulation, Appetite regulation	A-MSH, Vegf, Atm, Mdm2, Myc, Ccnd1, Ccna, Ifng	Loss of food anticipatory activity; cancer-prone, abnormal response to gamma irradiation, increased cellular proliferation; reduced muscular strength under stress; altered lipid metabolism, lower body weight, increased urinary sodium excretion, $Per2^{-/-}$ mice development obesity, increased bone density.
Cry	Liver, intestine	Xenobiotic detoxification, cell proliferation	Wee1, Cdk1, Cyp2e1, Hsd3b6	Impaired liver regulation; reduced a-adrenoceptor responsivense, salt sensitive hypertension; reduced tumor development, lowered incidence of cancer; hyperglycemia; Salt-sensitive hypertension
Rev-erbα	Adipose tissue, liver, serum, kidney	Adipocyte differentiation, Hepatic gluconeogenesis, Triglyceride catabolism	PPARγ2, ApoC-III, MTP	Elevated serum VLDL triglycerides; delayed proliferation and migration of granule cells; increased apoptosis of neurons in the internal granule cell layer;

Factor	Selected Tissue Distribution	Selected Physiology Roles	Selected Targets Genes	Phenotype of Knockout mice
Rorα	Skeletal muscle	Fatty acid oxidation Lipid homeostasis, several immune functions; steroids, bile acids and Xenobitotics mtabolism	Cpt1, Caveolin-3, ApoC-2, ApoA1,Cyp7b1, Srebf1,Fgf21, Pcp2, Pcp4,	Lower plasma triglyceride; abnormal lymphoid organ development, reduced survival rates of thymocytes, reduced susceptibility t autoimmune and inflammatory disorders, thin long bones; ataxia and severe cerebellar atrophy; reduced plasma triglycerides and HDL, enhanced atherosclerosis
PPARα	Liver and skeletal muscle	Lipid and energy metabolism; fatty acid oxidation and storage	Bmal1, Rev-erbα, ApoC-III	PPARα stimulates plasma Triglyceride clearance by stimulating LPL expression; decrease plasma Triglyceride, HDL; PPARα agonists down-regulate the expression of APOC3, ApoAC2, ApoA1, up-regulation the expression of ANGPLT4, LPL
PPARγ	Adipose, macrophage, liver	Fatty acid synthesis and storage in adipose tissues; Adipocytes differentiation	Rev-erbα	Lipid homeostasis
PGC1α	Liver, Skeletal muscle	Gluconeogenesis and energy metabolism	Bmal1, Rev-erbα	Increased sensitivity to insulin; Altered thermogenesis
FOXO1	Liver pancreatic	Embryonic vascular development	PGC1α; p27kip	Embryonic lethal (embryonic day 10.5) Defects of normal vascular development in embryo and yolk sac Lack of aortic arch vessels ; Hypoglycemia; lipid metabolism, liver-specific FOXO1 knockout mice caused a modest reduction in blood glucose concentrations and barely affected lipid homeostasis
Sirt1	Liver,	Cellular metabolism; lipid metabolism; cell growth, apoptosis, senescence, neuronal protection, adaptation to calorie restriction, organ metabolism	Clock (NPAS2)/Bmal1, PGC1α, PPARα, LXR, SREBP; ChREBP	Significant reduction in body weight. Liver Steatosis and Increased ChREBP Expression

Table 2. (Continued)

Factor	Selected tissue distribution	Selected physiology roles	Selected Targets, genes	Phenotype of Knockout mice
		and disease, DNA damage response and repair, and tumorigenesis		
Shp	Liver	Hepatic bile acid, lipid, and glucose homeostasis	PPARγ, SREBP-1c, CYP7A1, MTP, FAS	Increases in *CYP7A* 1, MTP mRNA; increased hepatic very-low-density lipoprotein (VLDL) secretion increase hepatic lipid accumulation
Nocturnin	Liver	A circadian deadenylase , lipogenesis, adipogenesis and osteogenesis; lipid metabolism	Srebp1a, Scd1, Fabpl, C/EBPα, Ppary2, aP2, Lpl. Ppary	Resistant to diet-induced obesity; altered lipid metabolism

In mammals the suprachiasmatic nucleus (SCN) of the hypothalamus region of the brain, there are an heterodimer of two transcription factors Bmal1 (also call brain and muscle ARNT-like 1) and Clock or a paralog of Clock, NPAS2 (neural period/ARNT/simpleminded 2) partner that positively controls the 24 hr circadian oscillatory period. Bmal1/Clock or Bmal1/NPAS2 together bind to E-box in promoter elements of target genes and activate transcription [17]. These targets include genes encoding Cry and Per proteins which also heterodimerize to directly repress Clock/Bmal1 feedback mechanism in the circadian oscillator; The Cry–Per complex directly inhibits Bmal1/Clock transcription, thereby ensuring a subsequent reduction in their own expression [17; 18]. As a consequence, the positive (Bmal1, Clock) and negative (Per, Cry) mRNAs are expressed in anti-phase to one another during a 24 hr period (Figure 1). Beside Clock and mTim, all Bmal1, Per1-3 as well as Cry1, 2 genes have shown different circadian rhythm in SCN (Table 1). Different Clock genes knockout mice have shown different phenotypes involving in triglyceride production and metabolism (Table 2).

2.2. Peripheral Oscillators

Results from several studies have indicated that peripheral oscillators have been demonstrated in different peripheral tissue, such as liver, heart, lung, kidney, as well as peripheral blood, within a 3 h- 9 h phase delay in oscillatory rhythms to compare their in the SCN phase [18]. Most peripheral Clock gene circadian rhythms have shown a phase delay relative to that in the SCN [18]. Knock out Clock gene can induce Bmal1 expression in peripheral tissues, but not in SCN [19-21], suggesting that Clock/Bmal1 heterodimers only can affects Bmal1 transcription level in the peripheral tissue.

Nevertheless, in 1998, the first paper on in vitro system published in cell appeared in volume 93 issue 6 [22]. The time when circadian rhythm research was difficult acceptance to most and searches for the circadian rhythm to regulate disease almost non-existent. In vitro cell culture experiment dates have indicated that cultures derived from peripheral tissue exhibit circadian rhythms which will be dampen after two to seven cycles, but not in SCN cells [22; 23]. These developments led the way to the development of circadian rhythm from in vivo system to in vitro system. These data also suggest that peripheral oscillators may involve a population of asynchronous cells requiring intermittent synchronizing stimuli, either from the SCN or from external entraining cues such as feeding.

The intestine is one of peripheral tissue to exhibit peripheral Clock. Clock genes are expressed in all regions of the intestine in rodents and mainly expression in enterocytes. The circadian oscillation of the conserved circadian mRNAs and proteins in the enterocytes of small intestine and their relation to lipid, protein, and macronutrient absorption in both wild-type and Clock mutant strains [24;29]. Furthermore, Clock mutant mice impacted the expression of critical nutrient transport proteins at the cellular level [24]. In addition, nocturn, a downstream target of Clock is responsible for mediating its effects in the small intestine [25]. We and other several research groups have indicated that Clock genes (Clock, Bmal1, Per1, Per2, Cry1, Cry2 as well as Reverbα, Reverbβ) have shown diurnal rhythm in all region of the intestine of rodents. These rhythm cycles are similar with the Clocks circadian rhythm of liver, but compared to the SCN, the phase are delay of approximately 6 h [24-28].

Animal studies by several groups have shown that transcription factors also shown significantly diurnal rhythm in small intestine similarly in the other tissues [7; 30; 31]. The Bmal1/Clock heterodimer also can directly bind E-box of their transcriptional targets factors such as the nuclear hormone receptor family members such as Rev-erbα (NR1D1), Rev-erbβ (NR1D2), Peroxisome proliferator-activated receptor (PPARs), retinoid-related orphan receptors (ROR)α, and RORβ, small heterodimer partner SHP (NROB2), the albumin D-site binding protein (DBP), and the leucine zipper protein E4BP4 (nuclear factor interleukin 3, NFIL3). These proteins also were called "Clock–

controlled genes" (CCGs), are controlled by Clock [18; 31]. Clock-control genes Rev-erbα proteins also serve as transcriptional repressors; they are counter-balanced by the transcriptional activation function of the ROR gene. DBP and E4BP4 also drive transcription from their own individual response element-specific circadian targets [31]. PPARγ directly regulates Bmal1 expression by interacting with cis elements at its promoter (Figure 1) [32]. Knockout of vascular PPPARγ significantly reduces the circadian rhythms in blood pressure and heart rate and is accompanied by impaired rhythmicity of Clock genes [32]. Liver-specific Bmal1 knockout mice abolished oscillations of plasma glucose and triglycerides levels [33].

Recently, a number of metabolic transcription factors and transcriptional co-activator factors have been shown to interact closely with circadian feedback loops (Table 2). On the other hand, Transcription factors can regulate circadian Clock, rendering the Clock responsive to numbers of factors including circulating hormones (cortisol, estrogen), nutrients sensors (fatty acids), calorie restriction, fasting, hypoxia and cellular redox condition (NADH/NAD+ ratio) [34].

The role of circadian Clocks was also described in the regulation of cancer diseases. Recent studies have revealed that Clock also play key parts in controlling metabolic homeostasis. Below, we discuss the functions of the Clock as well as Clock-controlled genes in triglyceride and lipid homeostasis physiological and therapeutic implications of these Clocks in metabolic diseases as illustrated in Figure 2.

3. Mutual Pathways of Dietary Triglyceride

3.1. Characteristic of Diurnal Rhythm of Intestinal and Liver Triglyceride *in Vivo*, in the Perfused Liver, Hepatocytes, Enterocytes, and in Cultured Cells

Few groups by wadhwa et al and raheja et al established that key features of triglycerides circadian rhythm in rat plasma and isolated liver as well as in younger and older chicks [35-37]. These works demonstrated that diurnal rhythm regulation of plasma triglyceride is: (*i*) rapid, occurring within 24 hrs; and (*ii*) sensitive to feeding and feeding compilation and (*iii*) plasma triglycerides decreased in controls between 0900 and 2100 hours and increased during the dark period. The forgotten implications of these landmark observations are that putative physiologic regulators of plasma triglyceride can be regulated at day and night by post-translational modifications of existing signaling complexes and by hormonal such as insulin, leptin, rather than by *de novo* gene transcription.

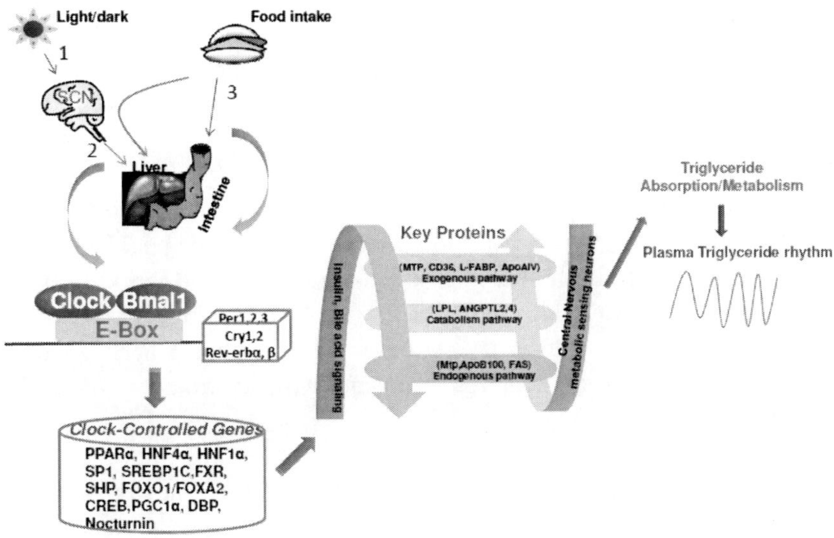

Figure 2. SCN-dependent pathway and Feeding-dependent pathway that both control peripheral Clocks genes regulate dietary triglyceride absorption and metabolism through activation of various signaling pathways. 1). Light entrainable oscillator through the retino-hypothalamic tract to the suprachiasmatic nuclei (SCN) in the brain, to changes various transcription factors that constitute the Clock genes. Circadian regulation in the SCN is crucially dependent on two transcription factors, Clock and Bmal1. Clock and Bmal1 heterodimers activate Per1, 2, 3 and Cry1, 2 genes, which heterodimerize to negatively regulate Clock/Bmal1 activity. **2).** The SCN master Clock phase-entrain peripheral Clocks through direct signaling pathway such as cyclic hormones insulin, Glucocorticoids and indirect pathways such as metabolism sensing neurons such as Fatty acid, and behavior feeding-fasting rhythm. **3).** Feeding rhythms are dominant over direct SCN synchronization cues of light-entrainable oscillator (LEO). When feeding rhythms are imposed upon and this will result in a turn over to push the phase of peripheral Clocks and uncouple it from the phase of the SCN pacemaker. For example, peripheral tissue Clock can be induced by 50% serum shock in human hepatocytes cell line (HepG2, Huh7 cell), however, SCN cell line could not induced by 50% serum shock. At the same gate, nervous system and hormones signaling as well as bile acid signaling are involving in the three pathways to regulate dietary triglyceride. Clock genes indirectly regulate key proteins of three pathway of dietary lipid such as diurnal regulation of MTP by Clock is mediated by Clock-controlled gene Shp.

In the 1980's, work in fed and fasted rats conclusively demonstrated that, one day fasting did not significantly affect the course of the *circadian* oscillations of rat plasma triglycerides and liver lipid metabolism in feeding condition, using cosinor analysis, this work emphasized the role of circadian Clocks [38]. The unintended consequence of this landmark research was that regulation of gene transcription and plasma triglyceride are all too often conflated into a single process, with recurring interpretive errors. Limited access to food studies have shown that limitation of the period for which they had access to food at different times of the day (from 8:30 am to 10:30 am, or 8:30 pm to 10:30 pm) significantly synchronized with the circadian oscillations of their serum and tissue lipid levels [39]. Much subsequent work has been stimulated by the finding that in rat, the peak of plasma triacylglycerol occurred 2 h after the beginning of the light period (7:00 am), and the nadir, 2 h after the beginning of the dark period (7:00 pm). The differences of plasma triglyceride at these two circadian stages were even more pronounced in food-deprived rats and were confined to the VLDL fraction [40].

Tracer studies in rats have defined circadian rhythm of triglyceride in detail, as in rats treated with triton WR1339, the amount of newly synthesized fatty acid secreted as VLDL triglyceride was greater during the dark phase of the diurnal cycle than during the light phase [40]. The liver cytosolic triglyceride content of the diabetic animals was significantly higher than normal at the mid-point of the dark phase of the cycle, and the diurnal variation was abolished in the diabetic animals [41].

In 1999, scientists have used of in vivo and in vitro techniques to study of the effects of insulin on hepatic triglyceride secretion in different insulinemic states [42]. Zammit et al determined that the effect of insulin on triglyceride secretion from rats under three metabolic conditions (insulin-deficient) fed normo-insulinaemic, 24-h fasted and fed, streptozotocin-diabetic by isolated perfused livers as well as in cultured hepatocytes [42].

Our several recent studies reported the discovery of the Clock expression in enterocytes as well as hepatocytes [24; 43]. Using a human "hemochromatotic" cell (Huh7) as well as *human liver hepatocellular carcinoma cell line* (HepG2) cells, we demonstrating that 50% horse serum induce circadian expression of small heterodimer partner (Shp), a Clock-controlled gene. In addition, a chaperon protein microsomal triglyceride transfer protein (MTP) mRNA and activity were augmented immediately after serum supplementation of Huh7 cells, also triglyceride secretion have shown a diurnal variation [24; 43]. Knock down Clock gene inhibit Shp to increased

MTP to boost intracellular triglyceride secretion in media of Huh7 cell as well as enterocytes [24; 43].

3.2. Regulation of Triglyceride in the Catabolism Pathway

In the mid 1980's, textbooks outlined the catabolism pathway by which diet lipid was hydrolyzed in the intestinal lumen through two step process. (i) Dietary triglyceride was break down physically in the mouth, stomach then solubilized in bile acid micelles in the intestinal duodenum and jejunum. (ii) Triglyceride molecules are digested into monoacylglycerols (MAG) and fatty acids by lipases/colipase. In these two process, several pancreatic lipases are required which include pancreatic triglyceride lipase, pancreatic triglyceride lipase related protein 2 and carboxyl ester lipase [44-46].

We know now that cell utilizes several enzyme mechanisms to clear up excess of triglycerides. The catabolism pathway needs to have normal lipoprotein lipase (LPL) activity. There are different half-lives of chylomicrons (CMs) and VLDLs, which are known about 10 minutes and 9 hours, respectively. And apo C-III, which inhibits LPL function, servicing for both exogenous and endogenous pathway triglyceride breakdown, is the conversion of triglyceride into free fatty acids and glycerol, free fatty acids are then stored in fat and muscle [45;46]. Due to the large size of unmetabolized CMs, they are unlikely to be taken up by macrophages, which are the precursors of foam cells, and then foam cells promote fatty streak formation and become the precursor of atherosclerotic plaque. LPL activity produces CM remnants that are small enough to take part in the atherosclerotic process [45;46]. LPL hydrolyzes triglycerides in both CMs and VLDL, releasing free fatty acids. The enzyme is found in the endothelial cells of capillaries and can be released into the plasma by heparin. LPL is essential for the metabolism of CMs and VLDL, transforming them into their respective remnants. Apo C-II, an apolipoprotein present in both CMs and VLDL, it acts as a cofactor in the action of LPL.

De et al have shown diurnal changes in LPL activity in heart and adipose tissue in rats fed a high and low fat diet [35], although they did not measured liver LPL account [35]. After 30 year later, Benavides et al demonstrated for the first time that LPL activities in plasma and various tissues, including liver, and HL activity in plasma follow circadian rhythms in wistar rats at physiological conditions [47]. The first of these observations in the rat was confirmed by in human test [48] and Dr. Gama research group made a commendable attempt to link LPL with diurnal rhythm in healthy volunteers [48]. However, additional work is necessary to dissect the significance of circadian rhythm in LPL catabolism pathway to regulate triglyceride. The mechanism of diurnal rhythm of LPL has not been reported to date. Although PPARα knockout mice have shown stimulates plasma TG clearance by stimulating LPL [49].

Angiopoietin-like (Angptl) 4 was found as a new member of the angiopoietin family. Human ANGPTL4 expression is ubiquitous with high expression in liver, adipose tissue, small intestine and heart [50]. ANGPTL4 are not only as a novel PPAR target in liver, but also as a novel target of PPARγ in adipose tissue [50]. Expression of the Angptl2 and Angptl4 genes exhibited 24-h rhythmicity [51; 52], which is similar to MTP diurnal rhythm. Serum Angptl2 levels were also found to show circadian expression and were reduced in db/db mice, circadian expression of Angptl2 in epididymal adipose tissue, reached a peak phase occurring at zeitgeber time (ZT) 12 [52].

ANGPTL3 and ANGPTL4 can inhibit LPL. Beside ANGPTL4, the recently elucidation of ANGPTL3 and glycosylphosphatidylinositol anchored high density lipoprotein binding protein 1 (GPIHBP1), which are also as major modulators of LPL function has underlined the complexity of the process of plasma triglyceride hydrolysis [50]. GPIHBP1 play important function as a stabilizer or even an anchor of LPL, which may neutralize ANGPTL3 and ANGPTL4-mediated LPL inhibitions [50]. However, the mechanisms still do not know. So far limited information is available about regulation of GPIHBP1 gene were recently found to be associated with severe hypertriglyceridemia and chylomicronemia in human [53]. Overexpression or deletion of ANGPTL4 in a variety of animal models has a stimulatory effect on plasma triglyceride levels, which is achieved by inhibiting LPL-dependent lipolysis of TG-rich lipoprotein. Similar result regulates plasma triglyceride by ANGPTL3 as compared to ANGPTL4, although presumably via different mechanisms [54]. In addition, PPARβ/δ is a potent inducer of ANGPTL4. PPARβ/δ suppresses ANGPTL3 expression. GPHBP1 expression is under control of PPARγ, albeit in different cell types [54; 55]. Taken together, these information revels an extensive and integrated network of functional interactions between the LPL and Clock controlled genes PPARs to regulate triglyceride and lipid homeostasis through the triglyceride catabolism pathway, although we still do not know whether Clock directly or indirectly regulate LPL. In the Bmal1$^{-/-}$ mice liver, a robust (78-fold) increase in LpL expression was observed [56].

3.3. Regulation of Triglyceride in the Exogenous Pathway

With the elucidation of the triglyceride pathway has come the realization that 10 of the 12 participating protein play multiple roles in the dietary lipid absorption and metabolism [57-59]. For example, at normal physiological condition, dietary lipids are hydrolyzed by in the lumen of the intestine and enterocytes absorb the products, then through two pathways (i) the lipids are re-synthesized by enterocytes and packaged into chylomicrons (CMs) a lipoprotein. (ii) The assembly of CMs occurs in the endoplasmic reticulum (ER) in a process requiring not only have a structural protein apoB48, but also need a dedicated chaperone protein MTP, which play the essential role of triglyceride production [60].

Another multiple of proteins act on both intermediates in the tag uptake and synthesis pathway such as plasma membrane fatty acid binding protein (FABPpm), fatty acid transport protein 4 (FATP4), and fatty acid translocase (FAT/CD36) and then free fatty acid is translocated to the endoplasmic reticulum (ER) by cytosolic fatty acid binding proteins (L-FABP and I-FABP) [57;59]. In addition, in the ER, three triglyceride synthesis proteins including Monoacylglycerol acyltransferase (MGAT) 2, diacylglycerol acyltransferase (DGAT) 1 as well as DGAT2 convert MAG and fatty acid to triglyceride [57]. Thus, the newly generated tag is transport with newly translated apoB48 is lipidated by MTP to form primordial CM that is further expanded in size by the addition of triglyceride in the core by MTP to form a pre-CM. These particles also acquire apoAIV at this step [61]. Prechylomicrons are concentrated and exported from the ER in prechylomicron transport vesicle (PCTVs). L-FABP facilitates the budding of PCTV from the ER. These vesicles then fuse with the cis-Golgi in a process that requires vesicle-associated membrane protein 7 (VAMP7). In the Golgi, apoA1 is added to prechylomicrons. Later, these particles are transported to plasma membrane using different transport vesicles and are ultimately released towards the basolateral side of enterocytes into circulation [62]. Triglyceride is exclusively transported via the CM pathway.

Physiological changes in feeding behavior show the 24-hours cycle, with a peak of food consumption occurring during the dark period associated with changes in various plasma parameters such as plasma triglycerides and cholesterol levels as well as ApoB48 [24;63]. In the intestine, CM assembly and secretion is a major mechanism for elimination of dietary lipid absorption, and MTP, shows distinct circadian expression [24; 63]. The circadian oscillation of the transport activity of MTP is synchronous with its mRNA level [63]. Furthermore, it was demonstrated that the circadian pattern of MTP activity is regulate by persisting under complete darkness, continuous illumination or fasting conditions [63]. Consistent with this, triglyceride absorption and enterocytes secretion of triglyceride, cholesterol exhibit distinct daily rhythms that are in accordance with the MTP rhythm [24]. ApoB gene expression has shown similarly diurnal rhythm. Disruption of this coordinately regulated pathway can result in the accumulation of triglyceride in the liver or hepatosteatosis [64]. A variety of common metabolic abnormalities such as obesity, diabetes and nonalcoholic fatty liver disease are associated with hepatosteatosis in both humans and animal models.

Similarly with MTP, intestinal apoAIV show a diurnal rhythmically released and the rhythm is controlled by the timing of meals, with levels increasing before meal onset [65; 66]. The serum apoAIV concentration also maintained a circadian rhythm and was high during the dark [65]. On the other hand, CD36 also can as small-intestinal lipid sensor, play a role throughout the oro-sensory reception of dietary lipids in the intestinal tract, shown a specific diurnal rhythms in mouse circumvallate papillae (CVP), *CD36* mRNA levels in CVP tended to be lower during the dark period than during the light period, shift with plasma lipid diurnal rhythm [67]. These observations suggest lipid-mediated down-regulation of CD36 protein.

At the same gate, under a normal LD cycle and mice with free access to food, DGAT2, and I-FABP mRNA showed diurnal variations [24], As well as the L-FABP mRNA level at the end of the light cycle (ZT16) transiently increased and thereafter decreased to near the original level after ZT22 [68].

The identification of the fatty acid synthesizing enzymes (FAS) and stearoyl CoA desaturase (SCD) 1 are showed a reciprocal diurnal expression pattern. SCD1 expression was high during the day, whereas FAS expression was high at night [24;69]. Nevertheless, both of these enzymes were significantly induced at mealtime [24]. These data indicate that some genes involved in triglyceride biosynthesis and secretion have diurnal variations. However, all the genes robustly respond to food entrainment.

While circadian Clock gens have been shown to regulate the rhythm of intestine lipid absorption, the role of other Clock genes is less well understood. Nocturnin is a circadian Clock-controlled gene, a downstream transcriptional mediator of the circadian Clock, which has equal importance to that of DBP, Rev-erbα, and ROR [18]. Knock out nocturnin can decrease CM transit into the plasma following the ingestion of dietary lipids [25]. *Noc*$^{-/-}$ mice absorb less triglyceride and cholesterol as compared to *Noc*$^{+/+}$ mice, similar results were found using isolated enterocytes [25].

Together, these studies demonstrate that nocturnin as an important regulator of intestinal CM processing, suggesting that the absence of nocturnin increases storage of lipids and decreases assembly and secretion of CM.

3.4. Regulation of Triglyceride in the Endogenous Pathway

The circadian Clock may play an important role in the liver physiology via regulation of fatty acid and glucose metabolism, and thus represent an important link between Clock and metabolism disorders such as obesity and fatty liver disease.

The Clock has previously been shown to regulate nuclear receptors such as liver X receptor (LXR), retinoid x receptor (RXR), PPARα and sterol response element binding proteins (SREBPs) in metabolic tissues and these receptors have play a role in cholesterol and fatty acid absorption and metabolism [70]. A number of Clock–controlled genes such as RORs, PPARs and tryroid hormone receptors (TRα) exhibit circadian rhythm in liver [71; 72] these proving a possible explanation for the diurnal rhythm in glucose and lipid metabolism.

Lipoprotein VLDL are taken up by the liver and assembled in the endoplasmic reticulum of hepatocytes [55]. Similar to that in the intestine, apoB100, triglyceride and phospholipids also form the surface of VLDL to regulate hepatocytes VLDL synthesis and secretion. Like the catabolism of CMs, the VLDL triglycerides are hydrolyzed by LpL, generating smaller and denser VLDL and subsequently intermediate-density lipoprotein (IDL) in the plasma. IDLs acquire apoE and are cleared fast from plasma only in minutes by hepatic receptors, LDL receptor (LDL-R) and LDL receptor-related protein (LRP), via receptor-mediated endocytosis [1; 73]. LDLs are cleared slowly approximately 48 h, relying on apoB100, which binds to the LDL-R in the liver. The assembly and secretion of VLDL is very complex and comprised substrates, hormones and neural signals [1; 73]. The liver VLDL assembly and secretion are involved in apoB100, MTP, fatty acid synthase (FAS), SREBP1c, and other protein.

MTP is play important role in the production of VLDL and its activation is also under control of transcription factors such as PPARα, hepaocyte nuclear factor (HNF4α, HNF1α), Specificity protein (Sp)1, SREBP1c, farnesoid X receptor (FXR) and Forkhead box (FOXO1/ FOXA2) in the liver [74].

Mutant Clock increase liver triglyceride accumulation in the liver, Clock/Bmal1/Npas2 enhances Shp expression and reduces MTP expression in the daytime to regulate plasma triglyceride [43]. High levels of Rev-erbα expression at night might suppress Shp expression and enhance MTP expression [43], suggest that not only Clock gene control liver MTP, but also Clock controlled gene Shp regulate MTP.

It is interesting to note that MTP is also targeted by other Clock, such as peroxisome proliferator activated receptor gamma coactivator 1 (PGC1α, PGC1β), which were also shown to modulate hepatocytes triglyceride, indicating that MTP regulation by Clock is likely to be complex.

Knock out Bmal1 can induced Cd36, FABP5, and scavenger receptor class B type I (Srbi) in the liver [75]. Fibroblast growth factor 21 (Fgf21) is a potent antidiabetic and triglyceride-lowering hormone whose hepatic expression is highly responsive to food intake and shown circadian rhythm [76;77]. Fgf21 was also recently shown to be a target of E4BP4, a key circadian output protein [78]. Expression of Fgf21 displays a circadian rhythm, which peaks during the fasting phase and is anti-phase to E4bp4, which is elevated during feeding periods. E4BP4 strongly suppresses Fgf21 transcription by binding to a D-box element in the distal promoter region [78]. E4BP4 is a novel insulin-responsive repressor of Fgf21 expression during circadian cycles and feeding [78]. In addition, Dr. Joseph bass group have shown that Clock mutant mice development metabolism syndrome, hyperlipidemia, hyperglycemia and fatty liver disease [79].

Recently, Per2 was found to play important role in liver through interactions with PPARα, HNF4α, TRα as well as Rev-erbα, although their direct involvement in the regulation of circadian rhythm has not been yet established [71;72].

4. Regulation of Triglyceride by Insulin, Bile Acid, AMPK, and c-AMP Signaling

4.1. Insulin Signaling Pathway

Several circadian Clocks have recently been implicated in controlling both lipids metabolism and insulin signaling and at multiple levels. Insulin is a hormone synthesized and secreted in pancreatic β-cells in response to increased nutrient levels and lipid metabolism in the blood, plasma insulin itself was shown diurnal rhythm and affect liver metabolism. Intestinal lipoprotein production is increased in both postabsorptive and postprandial states in an animal models of insulin resistance and type 2 diabetes [80;81], Some have proposed that CM production is acutely suppressed by insulin in chow-fed hamsters in vivo [82]; In insulin sensitive, intestinal lipoprotein production is responsive to the acute inhibitory effect of insulin [82]. This is consistent with increased intestinal lipoprotein production in insulin resistance and obesity in humans. Incubation of human fetal small intestinal cells with insulin reduces CM synthesis as well as secretion [83]. Not only in animal models, but also in healthy men, postprandial apoB 48 levels were correlated to insulin levels induced by ingestion of meals with varied glycemic index, while apoB48 levels were decreased during a 3 hour euglycemic, hyperinsulinemic clamp [83]. The precise mechanisms where by which insulin suppresses CM production remain poorly defined.

Some studies have determined that since elevated free fatty acid stimulates CM production, insulin may exert its effects on CM production through modulation of circulating free fatty acid levels [84]. However, Pavlic et al study showed that co-infusion of intra-lipid and heparin to prevent the insulin-mediated in vivo suppression of plasma free fatty acid only partially restored CM production during a euglycemia, hyperinsuinemic clamp in healthy humans, suggesting a role of insulin in regulating CM production beyond its modulation of free fatty acid [83]. This regulatory mechanism by insulin seems to be lost or diminished with impaired insulin responsiveness, thus insulin's ability to acutely inhibit CM production is blunted in T2D patients. In animal models, for example, *Psammomys obesus* insulin-resistant and diabetic sand rats contain increased amounts of L-FABP, higher MGAT and DGAT activities and show elevated apoB48 biogenesis. Insulin-resistant, sucrose-fed hamsters exhibit increased de novo lipogenesis, higher amounts of MTP and over production of apoB48 [85].

In addition to the functions of CM production by insulin, hepatic insulin resistance have been shown to affects lipid metabolism in vivo and in vitro such as perfused livers and cultured hepatocytes

The temporal or prolonged diurnal exposure of the liver to high basal insulin, to effect hepatic VLDL secretion, may explain the reason for the initial induction of muscle insulin resistance, under conditions generated by a Western- style pattern food. We went into detail explaining several factors such as FOXO1, PGC1α that will contribute to the regulation of plasma triglyceride in insulin-dependent pathway.

Forkhead-O Transcription Factors (FOXO1)

The PI-3 K/Akt/FOXO1or FOXA2 pathways have been shown a critical for insulin regulation of hepatic lipid metabolism [86-89]. For example, the main nuclear forkhead box O1 (FOXO1) targets, MTP and apoC-III, which both is catalyzing the rate-limiting steps in the production and clearance of triglyceride-rich lipoproteins [88; 89]. FOXO1 increases Akt signaling and suppresses PPPARα expression, leading to increased triglyceride synthesis and decreased fatty acid oxidation [86]. At the same time, the activity of FOXO1 is inhibited by insulin. FOXO1 can be deregulated, contributing to a liberated FOXO1 activity in the liver of in insulin resistant states. This effect contributes to hepatic overproduction of VLDL and impaired catabolism of triglyceride-rich particles, accounting for the pathogenesis of hypertriglyceridemia through MTP and apoC-III hepatic expression is inhibited by insulin [88; 89]. Similarly FOXO1, FOXA2 along with PGC-1β, also activates the expression of MTP and promotes apoB-containing VLDL secretion and is regulated by insulin [90]. Liver-specific FOXO1 knockout mice caused a modest reduction in blood glucose concentrations and barely affected lipid homeostasis [91].

Triglycerides are also formed in response to fluxes of free or unsaturated fatty acids and glucose. Glucose can indirectly provide de novo lipogenesis, through pyruvate citrate generating acetyl-CoA for fatty acid synthesis [92]. Some data suggest that feeding high-carbohydrate meal activates lipogenesis by insulin activation of SREBP1c [92].

PGC1α

Aside from their indirect involvement in the diurnal regulation of plasma triglyceride machinery, the peroxisome proliferator-activated receptor g coactivator-1 (PGC-1) family of transcriptional coactivators is emerging as a center linking lipid and hormonal signals pathway.

PGC-1α is expressed in pancreatic β-cells, PGC-1α is also involved in insulin pathway, fasting can induce liver PGC1α gene expression through glucagon and glucocorticoid (GR) signaling [93], PGC-1α has the ability to increase the transcriptional activity of many nuclear receptor families, such as members of the estrogen, PPAR, glucocorticoid receptor (GR), liver X (LXR), and thyroid hormone receptor families [94]. PGC-1α can also bind to nuclear hormone receptors including HNF4α, FXR, PPARα and ERRα [94], suggesting that their conformations are conductive to ligand-independent mechanisms of gene regulation. Further, it is now evident that PGC-1 α is a key component of the circadian oscillator that integrates the peripheral Clock and energy metabolism [95-98]. PGC-1α can stimulate the expression of Bmal1 through coactivation of the ROR family of orphan nuclear receptors in peripheral tissue hepatocytes and muscle cells [99;100].

PGC1 family is also has been implicated in promoting transcription of lipid proteins. Specifically, PGC-1β plays an important role in plasma lipoprotein homeostasis [90]. Again, several factors are involved in mediating the effects of PGC-1β on plasma triglyceride metabolism, including SREBP1c, LXR, and FoxA2. In vitro experiment suggests that peroxisome proliferator-activated receptor alpha-RXRalpha and PGC-1β coordinately up-regulate L-FABP and MTP expression [90]. Hepatic-specific PGC1α knockout mice accumulate triglyceride in liver, due to impaired β-oxidation, and enhanced SREBP1c-stimulated fatty acid and triglyceride synthesis [91].

A recent study revealed that circadian Clock play critical role in proliferation and function of pancreatic β cells. As mentioned above, mice with mutation Clock gene are obese and develop a metabolic syndrome consisting of hyperleptinemia, hyperlipidemia, and hyperglycemia [79]. Loss of Bmal1gene leads to uncoupling and impaired glucose-stimulated insulin secretion in β-cells [101]. In addition, $Bmal1^{-/-}$ knockout mice, similarly to Clock mutant mice, exhibited suppressed diurnal rhythm in glucose and triglyceride as well as abolished gluconeogenesis [101].

Taken together, these results reveal an extensive and integrated network of functional interactions between the liver nuclear transcription factors and their Clock to regulate triglyceride and lipid homeostasis [102]. As noted above, the mechanisms underlying this complex metabolic disease remain to be fully elucidated in increase number of Clock have now been implicated in the control of insulin signaling and glucose homeostasis at all steps of regulation, from pancreatic islet development, β-cell differentiation and insulin secretion to target tissue insulin sensitivity and intracellular insulin signaling to downstream effectors.

These findings indicate that Clock play a role in controlling liver lipid metabolism through effects on nuclear transcription factors and insulin signal pathways.

4.2. Bile Acid Signaling

The last two decades have witnessed the bile acid which are produced by hepatocytes and secreted with cholesterol, phospholipids and other part as bile fluid in the bile canaliculi of the liver. In the liver-gut bile acid cycle processing, bile acid are transported into the enterocytes by bile acid transporters, and then transferred into the portal vein for return to the liver [103]. In rodents, the direct effects of bile acid in intestine are necessary, but not sufficient to inhibit triglyceride absorption.

Several recent studies reported the discovery of the bile diversion which abolishes the circadian rhythm of lymph flow, lymph apoAIV, triglyceride, and cholesterol, suggesting that bile acid was an important determinant of their circadian rhythm [65]. Bile acid levels ensure appropriate cholesterol catabolism, and promote optimal solubilization and absorption of fat and other essential nutrients. Bile acid can activate nuclear receptors such as FXR [104]. Recent studies have indeed demonstrated that FXR and FXR downstream targets such as SHP play a key role in the control of hepatic de novo lipogenesis, VLDL-triglyceride export and plasma triglyceride turnover [105]. REV-ERBα is a key player in the circadian regulation of cholesterol and bile acid synthesis by influencing rhythmic SREBP activity and cholesterol 7-alpha-monooxygenase or cytochrome P450 7A1 (*CYP7A1)* expression [106]. FXR indirectly inhibits CYP7A1 expression through inducing expression of FGF15 [107]. The CYP7A1and FGF15 in both the cholesterol and bile acid metabolic pathway has long been known to show distinct circadian variation in their expression level and enzymatic activity [108-113].

CYP7A1 are induced by SHP in mice as well as by the HNF4α [107]. CYP7A1 mRNA levels and activity show strong diurnal variation [111]. CYP7A1 expression was recently found to be under the control of the DBP, Dec2 (also called Stra13 or Sharp-2), and E4BP4, which are Clock control genes [111].

In the intestine, the FXR target gene SHP encodes an atypical orphan nuclear receptor that was believer to lacks a DNA binding domain and represses expression of MTP genes implicated in triglyceride [43]. Our group have shown that Shp shown significantly diurnal rhythm, high in day time, low in the midnight [43], Shp knockout mice show modest fed and fasted hyperglycemia and at same time resistance to bile acid inhibition of Glucose-6-phosphatase (G6pc) and Phosphoenolpyruvate carboxykinase 1 (Pck1) as well as induced plasma triglyceride through to induced MTP [43;114]. Conversely, SHP overexpression by injected adenoviruses in liver reduced MTP expression and lowered plasma triglyceride in Clock mutant mice [43]. Interestingly, Shp is negatively regulated by Rev-erbα, as siRev-erbα was also found to decreases MTP expression in Huh-7 cells, mutant Clock *increase* MTP gene expression, decrease levels of Rev-erbα, both MTP and Rev-erbα do not show temporal changes in *Clock* mution mice, both Rev -erbα and MTP show peak expression at similar times [43]. Therefore, it is likely that Rev-erbα indirectly regulates MTP via Shp [43]. it may additionally affect of bile acid signaling intermediate MTP through both the positive and negative loops of the circadian Clock are involved in the diurnal regulation of MTP Clock/Bmal1/Npas2 enhance Shp expression and reduce MTP expression in the daytime. High levels of Rev-erbα expression at night might suppress Shp expression and enhance Mtp expression at night [43]. Recently, Rev-erbα was found to play an important role in the control of bile acid metabolism via the regulation of the neutral bile acid synthesis pathway [115;116]. In addition, Rev-erbα also controls the daily expression of genes involved in cholesterol and lipid homeostasis through circadian modulation of SREBP signaling [115; 116]. Rev-erbα knockout mice have shown that elevated serum VLDL triglycerides; delayed proliferation and migration of granule cells; increased apoptosis of neurons in the internal granule cell layer [117];

In addition to the FXR or Rev-erbα transcriptional mechanism, bile acids may also inhibit VLDL production independent of FXR. FXR may regulate lipogenesis also independently of SREBP1c by enhancing FAS transcription. Other way to decrease triglyceride by FXR are due to PPARα activation, which promotes FFA catabolism through activation of pyruvate dehydrogenate kinase-4 (PDK-4) [118]. FXR also activity lipolysis by activating apoC-II, through stimulates LPL activity, and decrease apoC-III and ANGPTL3 [119].

These results raise the interesting possibility that disruption of bile acid homeostasis and the resultant accumulation of bile acids in the liver might be important in the absorption of lipid that have long been among the best known health complications of shift work.

Taken together, these results reveal an extensive and integrated network of functional interactions between the transcription factors as circadian rhythm control genes such as Shp, DBP, E4BP4 and triglyceride production and catabolism key factors genes such as LPL, MTP that regulate triglyceride diurnal rhythm and lipid homeostasis by circadian rhythm control genes Rev-erbα through bile acid pathway.

4.3. AMPK Signaling -role of Clock in Hepatic Steatosis Management

Loss of circadian rhythm in Clock mutant mice exhibited not only attenuated diurnal feeding rhythm, hyperphagia, obsity and development a metabolic syndrome of hyperliptinemia, hyperglycemia hyperlipidemia but also induce hepatic steatosis [79]. As mentioned above, several studies have measured Clock regulation liver metabolism could affect other key metabolic targets of Clock, such as NAD-dependent deacetylase sirtuin-1 (SIRT1), SREBPs, PPARs, PGC1α, LXR and FOXO1, potentially further contributing to hepatosteatosis [120]. Sirtl KO mice have shown that significant reduction in body weight induces liver Steatosis and Increased ChREBP Expression [121].

It is well known that nonalcoholic and alcoholic fatty liver each begin resulting from the accumulation of lipids in the liver. Lipid accumulation in the liver which induces hepatic steatosis can occur through four different pathways:

(1) Maladaptations of fatty acid uptake, it can explain that fatty acid uptake through both dietary uptake and lipolysis in adipose tissue can contribute to the pathogenesis of both disorders, as can effects on fatty acid transporters, such as CD36.
(2) Fatty acid synthesis, fatty acid synthesis in alcoholic and nonalcoholic fatty liver are involve the endoplasmic reticulum (ER) stress response, homocysteine metabolism pathway, and different transcription factors regulating genes in the lipid synthesis pathway.
(3) Fatty acid oxidation, fatty acid oxidation, through effects on AMP-activated protein kinase (AMPK), adiponectin, PPARs, and mitochondrial function is predominantly altered in alcoholic liver disease, although studies suggest that activation of this pathway may improve nonalcoholic fatty liver disease. Activation of AMPK results in enhanced fatty acid oxidation and decreased production of glucose, cholesterol, and triglycerides.
(4) Export of lipids from the liver. Changes in fatty acid export, through effects on apoB and MTP are seen in both diseases. Thus, the similarities and differences in the mechanism of fat accumulation in the liver in nonalcoholic and alcoholic liver disease are explored in detail.

Now, hepatic steatosis is understood to play an important role in the development of advanced liver disease. The circadian Clock plays an important role in regulating these processes in a temporal manner. There are the two important signalings for lipid homeostasis, insulin and AMPK [120]. As aforementioned, insulin inhibit FOXO1 or FOXA2 decrease MTP to accumulation triglyceride in the liver. Insulin has the opposite effect. AMPK is a crucial energy sensor of the AMP/ATP ratio. AMPK is as also Clock-associated enzymes protein. The circadian rhythm regulation of the SIRT1-PGC1α pathway is at least partially dependent on AMPK in vivo [120]. AMPK is as a fuel gauge by sensing increased AMP/ATP ratio, as a cellular sensor of energy level [120]. AMPK activity stimulates food intake in the hypothalamus AMPK activity also stimulates fatty acid uptake and oxidation in the periphery [120;122]. AMPK has a diurnal rhythm in hypothalamu, and is a essential for circadian rhythm generation in mouse embryonic fibroblasts [123-125]. AMPK may transmit nutrient signals directly to the Clock by the intermediate player Cry1 and Per2 [123-125]. For example, AMPK induces a phase advance of circadian expression of Clock genes by degrading PER2 through phosphorylating Casein kinase Iε Ser389 in peripheral tissues [126], and AMPK has been found to phosphorylating and destabilizing Cry1 [125] and instead increasing its binding to F-box and Leu-rich repeat protein 3 (FBXL3), a ubiquitin ligase that promotes Cry1 ubiquitylation and degradation. In addition, the circadian rhythm of Clock genes is absent in AMPKα1/α2$^{-/-}$ in mouse embryonic fibroblasts [123].

It has been known for many years that the phosphorylation of AMPK targets acetyl CoA carboxylase (ACC) following a circadian rhythm in rodent liver under food intake [127]. The more recent studies suggest that AMPK may have a crucial role in determining these circadian rhythms.

AMPK promotes fatty acid uptake into cardiac myocytes via translocation of vesicles containing the fatty acid transporter CD36 to the plasma membrane. Transcriptional control by AMPK may be important for the treatment of liver steatosis because AMPK activation suppresses expression of SREBP1c [128; 129].

Therefore, the circadian Clock regulates AMPK activity to fulfill the liver triglyceride metabolism during the diurnal physiological cycles. In addition, various metabolic energy states also regulate AMPK activity and influence the circadian rhythm by controlling the degradation of Per2 and Cry1.

All in all, the information made on the effecting of AMPK on circadian Clock gene expression render AMPK a probable regulator for coupling circadian Clock to triglyceride metabolism cycles.

4.4. c-AMP Signaling (CREB)

An important pathway through which the circadian rhythm Clock controlled gene Cyclic-AMP-responsive-element-binding protein (CREB) may modify lipid metabolism responses is the CREBH pathway [130]. CREBH is a transcription factor that is highly and selectively expressed in liver and small intestine. Several recent studies suggest that hepatic CREBH is transcriptional activated by fasting, and induce lipid metabolism genes, including in apoAIV, apoAV, and apoC-II which exhibit stimulatory effects on LPL [130]. CREBH knockout mice showed hypertriglyceridemia, associated with defective production of these apolipoproteins and decreased LPL activity [131].

5. Direct and Indirect Mechanisms

We now know that the Clock transcription factor system located in the SCN of the brain hypothalamus, acts as the "master" oscillator and generator of the body's circadian rhythm under the strong influence of the light/dark input from the eyes [132]. The peripheral Clock system distributed in all organs and tissues, including the central nervous system (CNS) outside the SCN, acts generally as a "slave" Clock under the regulation of the central SCN Clock by as yet unknown mechanisms; both neuronal and hormonal connections have been implicated [9;132;133].

The central Clock under the regulation of the light input controls and overrides the hypothalamic-pituitary-adrenal (HPA) axis, which signals from the brain trigger the release of hormones needed to respond to stress, and produces regular diurnal secretion of glucocorticoid hormones from the adrenal glands, while the peripheral Clock genes, which are located in the adrenal glands and other components of the HPA axis and are regulated by the central Clock through neural and humoral pathways, also contribute to the rhythmic glucocorticoid secretion from these organs [134;135]. Secreted glucocorticoid can in turn reset and phase-delay circadian rhythm of the peripheral Clock genes by stimulating the expression of several Clock-related genes [134; 135]. The peripheral Clock genes also regulate glucocorticoid effect in local tissues through interaction between Clock/Bmal1 and GR, providing a local counter regulatory feedback loop to the effect of central Clock on the HPA axis [136]. The Circadian Clock may integrate information obtained from several tissues and organs via both humoral and neuronal pathways.

5.1. Food Intake -as an Output and Input System of Circadian Clock System

During the past decade, a growing amount of evidence indicates that gut-brain axis is a key partner of lipid homeostasis. Both afferent nerves and gastrointestinal hormones are the link between the periphery and the brain. Molecules such as insulin, leptin, and *Glucagon-like peptide-1* (GLP-1) have emerged as key factors able to convey metabolic information to the brain and also to modulate endogenous triglyceride absorption and metabolism.

Food intake is responsible for the major increase in intestine and liver triglyceride during the circadian cycle. However, fasted rat still showed plasma triglyceride circadian rhythms, indicating that an entrainable oscillator controls changes in plasma triglycerides [38].

There are two pathways of light-entrainable and food-entrainable are major components of mammalian circadian timekeeping system. Food intake is coupled to the circadian Clock system as both an output and an input. Food intake can act as entrainment stimuli to controlling the phase and period of circadian Clock in the brain and peripheral organs and tissues such as intestine and liver. Peripheral organs and tissue contain food entrainable circadian oscillators; communicate with the brain by endocrine and neural signals [7]. Food is a potent synchronizer of peripheral Clocks and entrains various behavioral and physiologic activities. However, it is unknown whether food-entrainable work alone or there is significant cooperation between light-entrainable and food-entrainable during food entrainment. It is known that ablation of *Per1* and *Bmal1*, abolishes food entrainment [7;137-143]. We, using Clock mutant mice to study light- and food-entrained regulation of Clock and intestinal genes as well as absorptive functions of the gut [24]. Our data show that intestinal epithelial cells express canonical Clock genes in a circadian manner and are susceptible to attunement by food. Normal Clock expression is important for the circadian and food-entrained expression of nutrient transport proteins as well as in the absorption of triglyceride, cholesterol as well as glucose [24]. In addition to the liver and fat tissue, the intestine is a target tissue of the food-entrainable. The expressions of intestinal Clock genes were resistant to food entrainment in Clock mutant mice [24]. Hence, we propose that Clock is important for light and food entrainment of intestinal Clock genes.

However, a mechanism or mechanisms entraining peripheral tissues by the food-entrainable have not yet been elucidated. Although it was believed that glucocorticoid as well as AMPK played a part, as discussion above, it is now thought that glucocorticoid rhythm driven by the SCN opposes the food-entrainable response [144]. Instead, it has been hypothesized that circulating macronutrients and consequent activation of signaling pathways might be involved in resetting peripheral Clocks during food entrainment. This hypothesis places enormous importance on the intestine and macronutrient absorption as a signal for the entrainment of peripheral Clocks by food and warrants further research towards elucidating the role of the intestine in food entrained regulation of behavioral activities, physiologic processes and molecular events.

5.2. Central Nervous System Effects on Plasma Triglyceride in Rodents

The interconnection between circadian Clocks and lipid absorption and metabolism is also underscored by work on other model organisms. For example, rat jejunal vagal afferents are activated by infusions of lipid and fatty acids, such as intralipid and oleic acid [145].

Indeed, it is likely that lipids might directly or indirectly exert an effect on vagal afferents through three pathways: One is direct activation by CMs [145]; Secondly, CM-induced release of other activating substances, such as apoAIV [146]; Three, release of serotonin and actions on vagal serotonin 3 (5-HT_3) receptors located on primary vagal afferents [147]. The ability of intestinal lipid infusions to inhibit food intake and activate brain stem NTS c-fos is blocked by administration ondansetron, a selective 5-HT3 receptor antagonist. It is suggested that 5-HT3 receptors mediate gut vagal afferent signaling [147].

5.3. "Metabolic Sensing" Neurons: Fatty Acids, Leptin

Many neurons respond to a variety of metabolites and hormones from the periphery which informs them on the metabolic status of the body. In the jejunal vagal afferents, they are called "metabolic sensing neurons". "Metabolic sensing" neurons can respond to differences in the metabolic states related with feeding and fasting. For example, glucosesing neurons, which utilize glucose as a signaling molecule, were responsiveness to oleic acid (OA) dependent upon glucose concentrations [145; 148]. These specialized "metabolic sensing neurons", which were responsive to both OA and glucose [149], might show differentiate regulation between the fasted and fed states.

Similarly glycosensing neurons, exogenous fatty acids also can play as "metabolic sensing neurons" role in multiple signaling. Hypothalamic neurons can responsive to very low concentrations of fatty acids [148]. Each of these fatty acids probably plays an important role in neurons as building blocks for membranes and organelles [150].

Some studies also have shown that CD36 mRNA is expressed in ventromedial hypothalamic nucleus (VMN) neurons and that the responses of VMN neurons to OA occurred at concentrations that are close to the affinity constant for binding of fatty acids to CD36 [148]. Gut vagal afferents also contribute to the ability of oleoylethanolamide (OEA) to reduce feeding, as vagal capsaicin application blocks OEA induced satiety [151]. OEA an endogenous ligand for PPARα is diurnally regulated by food intake [152]. PPARs are known to regulate the transcription of both Bmal1 and Rev-erbα by interacting with the peroxisome proliferator response elements (PPREs) at their promoters [153]. OEA can increase CD36 expression in small intestinal enterocytes by exogenous administration of OEA, an endogenously produced fatty acid ethanolamide concentrated in duodenum and jejunum [154]. Probably nutritional lipid is translocated into the luminal tissue, stimulating gut OEA or/and oleic acid biosynthesis, which individually and/or together inhibit gut CD36 and PPAR alpha expression.

In addition, hormones such as leptin and insulin, these may have these same metabolic sensing neurons response, and vary markedly between the fed and fasted states [155]. Therefore providing additional inputs from the periphery to regulate the meal-related activity of ventromedial hypothalamic nucleus (VMN) neurons involved in the regulation of both energy homeostasis.

Surgical and chemical blockade of vagal efferent outflow to the intestine in wild-type mice failed to alter the triglyceride phenotype, demonstrating that central neural control mechanisms were likely not involved in the observed regulation of intestinal MTP [156]. Instead of vagal efferent, there are two types of leptin-responsive neurons, orexigenic neuropeptide Y/agouti gene related peptide (NPY/AGRP) neurons and anorexigenic proopiomel-anocortin/cocaine amphetamine regulated transcript (POMC/CART) neurons, the data shown that leptin receptor (LEPR) B and melanocortin 4 receptor (MC4R) may regulates intestinal MTP and controls intestinal lipid absorption [156].

Whether neuronal control of plasma triglyceride diurnal rhythm is unique to rodents remains disputed. Using a drosophila model of insomnia have elevated that dopamine are short-lived, and show increased levels of triglycerides, cholesterol, and free fatty acids. However, their core molecular Clock remains intact [157].

5.4. Arginine Vasopressin (AVP) Receptor Couples Metabolism with Circadian Rhythm

In addition to "Metabolic sensing" neurons, vasopressin is implicated in regulations of the blood osmosis and pressure. It is known that AVP is produced not only in the SCN, but also in the paraventricular nucleus (PVN) and the supraoptic nucleus (SN), and AVP in both PVN and SN are transported to the neurohypophysis via neural axons. AVP injected peripherally do not act on the hypothalamic thermoregulatory center but act on the peripheral metabolic tissues [158].

Studies have shown that AVP-induced hypothermia and the suppression of lipolysis can modulate the lipid metabolism in brown adipose tissue by reducing sympathetic nervous activity [159].

AVP-induced reduction in body temperature was caused by a reduction in the metabolic rate associated with the suppression of the lipid metabolism [158]. In fasting condition, knock down Vasopressin (AVP) receptor decrease serum triglyceride. vasopressin receptor-deficient ($V1aR^{-/-}$) mice can increase serum triglyceride as well as cholesterol under feed condition [158], these effect might be due to increased insulin sensitivity that could cause a decreased in leptin levels, leading to suppressed lipolysis in $V1aR^{-/-}$ mice [158].

These suggest that AVP may integrate many signals at various cellular pathways related to Clock and lipid metabolism. However, it is not yet clear to what extent imposed Clock reflect the physiology of AVP to control lipid metabolism during normal feeding or fasting cycles in animal fed ad libitum.

5.5. Glucocorticoids -Crosstalk between Circadian Clock and Glucocorticoids in Regulation Triglyceride Absorption and Metabolism

In addition to AVP, other sensing rhythmic metabolic signals pathway such as Glucocorticoids (GCs) may also regulate lipid metabolism by circadian Clock. GCs hormones are major endocrine outputs of the Clock, playing major roles as mediators of temporal communication between the SCN and peripheral tissue [160; 161]. Clock/Bmal1 physically interacts with the ligand-binding domain of the GCs to suppress GCs-induced transcriptional activity through acetylation [162].

GCs are secreted by the adrenal gland. Circulating GCs display a strong diurnal rhythm that is controlled by the central Clock, in HPA axis of SCN in dependent fashion by altering the sensitivity of the adrenal cortex to Adrenocorticotropic hormone (ACTH) via SCN mediated activation of the autonomic nervous system [162;163]. Another possible is that the peripheral CLOCK located in the adrenal glands gates glucocorticoid production stimulated by fluctuating plasma ACTH. GCs bind to glucocorticoid response elements in Per1 and Per2 genes to regulate their rhythmic expression [162; 164].

GCs are a causative factor in many of the pathologies associated with diabetes, including hyperlipidemia and hyperglycemia. For example, chronically increased GCs result in hepatic lipid accumulation. Treatment of adrenalectomized mice with an exogenous glucocorticoid (dexamethasone) has been shown to induce expression of the apoAIV gene in adrenalectomized mice [165].

GCs were necessary for the stimulation of hepatic triglyceride production [166], and directly stimulate hepatic fatty acid, triglyceride synthesis, and to increase apoB secretion in hepatocytes [167; 168]. Recently, studies have shown that 11β-hydroxysteroid dehydrogenase type 1 (11β-HSD1) is an $NADP^+$/NADPH-dependent oxidoreductase that also can direction inactive 11-keto derivatives to active glucocorticoids to regulate plasma triglyceride in controversial areas [169], suggesting potential interactions between Clock and lipid metabolism through GCs, or GCs metabolism-related genes such as PPARr, which is part of the Clock controlled genes. Glucocorticoids have also been known to cause increases in apoAI expression levels through an unknown indirect mechanism [170; 171].

In the past few years, significant progress has been made in understanding the roles of the circadian Clock and GCs in regulating lipid metabolism and circadian rhythm.

6. Future Prospects

Major blank in our understanding of circadian control of triglyceride metabolism still remain. First, how does the nutritional state, hormonal as well as nervous and circadian Clock connect to control lipid metabolism? Second, since it is unlikely that Clock is the sole mediator of all Clock–control genes transcription factors such as Srebp1c, FOXO1, Shp and downstream genes such as Cyp7A1, MTP, CD36, which are the other Clock–uncontrolled genes protein partners in the epigenetic control of triglyceride metabolism? Third, what is the impact of the Clock (and Clock disorders) on human (patho) physiology, and, in particular, on cardiovascular diseases? Fourth, what is the inflammatory function in these processes to control lipid absorption as well as metabolism? Future studies should also address the question whether pharmacological modulation of Clock, Clock control genes as well as Clock relationship genes may provide a means to improve circadian disorder-related metabolic and cardiovascular dysfunctions.

CONCLUSION

Several important conclusions can be drawn about the link between the circadian Clock and triglyceride absorption and metabolism in the intestine and liver. 1) Plasma triglyceride is regulated by center and peripheral tissues circadian Clocks through neuronal, hormonal connections and molecular mechanism levels. 2) Reduced ileal absorption of bile acids leads to enhanced VLDL production, which links Clock to bile acid metabolism to regulate triglyceride production. 3) Circadian Clocks also contribute to insulin signaling and glucose homeostasis and highlight the potential pathological roles of aberrant Clocks expression in cardiometabolic disorders. 4) Hepatic Clock genes modulate both bile acid and apolipoprotein biosynthesis, raising the possibility that Clock disruption may impact multiple components of hepatic lipid homeostasis. For example, several proteins involved in lipid metabolism (such as CYP7A1, ANGPTL2, ApoA IV or MTP) show diurnal variation in humans and/or rodents. We discussed the role of Clock system in intestine and liver function. Key biochemical, cellular, and integrated physiological mechanisms by which circadian Clock regulate triglyceride have been clarified in this chapter.

ACKNOWLEDGMENTS

I am sincerely and heartily grateful to my mentor, Professor Mahmood Hussain, for his thoughtful guidance, academic advice, and warm encouragement. Also, I would like to thank to Dr Ahmed Bakillah for help reading and useful discussions of chapter. I would like to apologize to authors whose works were omitted owing to space limitations. I regret that I am unable to credit all contributors to this field. This work was supported in part by Scientist Development Grant (2300158) from AHA to X.P.

REFERENCES

[1] Hassing, H. C., Surendran, R. P., Mooij, H. L., Stroes, E. S., Nieuwdorp, M., and linga-Thie, G. M. (2012) *Biochim. Biophys. Acta* 1821, 826-832.

[2] Brewer, H. B., Jr. (1999) *Am. J. Cardiol.* 83, 3F-12F.

[3] Furman, A., Meier, J. L., Malmstrom, R. A., Lopez, J. R., and Schaefer, S. (2011) *Am. J. Manag. Care* 17, 538-544.

[4] Miller, M., Stone, N. J., Ballantyne, C., Bittner, V., Criqui, M. H., Ginsberg, H. N., Goldberg, A. C., Howard, W. J., Jacobson, M. S., Kris-Etherton, P. M., Lennie, T. A., Levi, M., Mazzone, T., and Pennathur, S. (2011) *Circulation* 123, 2292-2333.

[5] Brunner, D., Altman, S., Loebl, K., Schwartz, S., and Levin, S. (1977) *Atherosclerosis* 28, 197-204.

[6] Reardon, M. F., Nestel, P. J., Craig, I. H., and Harper, R. W. (1985) *Circulation* 71, 881-888.

[7] Hussain, M. M. and Pan, X. (2009) *Trends Endocrinol. Metab* 20, 177-185.

[8] King, D. P. and Takahashi, J. S. (2000) *Annu. Rev. Neurosci.* 23, 713-742.

[9] Takahashi, J. S. (1991) *Curr. Opin. Neurobiol.* 1, 556-561.

[10] Takahashi, J. S. (1993) *Curr. Opin. Genet. Dev.* 3, 301-309.

[11] Roldan, G. and Ang, R. C. (2006) *Respir. Care Clin. N. Am.* 12, 31-54, viii.

[12] Vitaterna, M. H., King, D. P., Chang, A. M., Kornhauser, J. M., Lowrey, P. L., McDonald, J. D., Dove, W. F., Pinto, L. H., Turek, F. W., and Takahashi, J. S. (1994) *Science* 264, 719-725.

[13] King, D. P., Zhao, Y., Sangoram, A. M., Wilsbacher, L. D., Tanaka, M., Antoch, M. P., Steeves, T. D., Vitaterna, M. H., Kornhauser, J. M., Lowrey, P. L., Turek, F. W., and Takahashi, J. S. (1997) *Cell* 89, 641-653.

[14] Forbes-Robertson, S., Dudley, E., Vadgama, P., Cook, C., Drawer, S., and Kilduff, L. (2012) *Sports Med.* 42, 185-208.
[15] Chong, S. Y., Ptacek, L. J., and Fu, Y. H. (2012) *Trends Genet.*
[16] Panda, S., Hogenesch, J. B., and Kay, S. A. (2003) *Novartis. Found. Symp.* 253, 73-82.
[17] Darlington, T. K., Wager-Smith, K., Ceriani, M. F., Staknis, D., Gekakis, N., Steeves, T. D., Weitz, C. J., Takahashi, J. S., and Kay, S. A. (1998) *Science* 280, 1599-1603.
[18] Green, C. B., Takahashi, J. S., and Bass, J. (2008) *Cell* 134, 728-742.
[19] DeBruyne, J. P., Noton, E., Lambert, C. M., Maywood, E. S., Weaver, D. R., and Reppert, S. M. (2006) *Neuron* 50, 465-477.
[20] DeBruyne, J. P., Weaver, D. R., and Reppert, S. M. (2007) *Nat. Neurosci.* 10, 543-545.
[21] DeBruyne, J. P., Weaver, D. R., and Reppert, S. M. (2007) *Curr. Biol.* 17, R538-R539.
[22] Balsalobre, A., Damiola, F., and Schibler, U. (1998) *Cell* 93, 929-937.
[23] Balsalobre, A., Marcacci, L., and Schibler, U. (2000) *Curr. Biol.* 10, 1291-1294.
[24] Pan, X. and Hussain, M. M. (2009) *J. Lipid Res.* 50, 1800-1813.
[25] Douris, N., Kojima, S., Pan, X., Lerch-Gaggl, A. F., Duong, S. Q., Hussain, M. M., and Green, C. B. (2011) *Curr. Biol.* 21, 1347-1355.
[26] Sladek, M., Rybova, M., Jindrakova, Z., Zemanova, Z., Polidarova, L., Mrnka, L., O'neill, J., Pacha, J., and Sumova, A. (2007) *Gastroenterology* 133, 1240-1249.
[27] Hoogerwerf, W. A. (2006) *Curr. Gastroenterol. Rep.* 8, 353-359.
[28] Hoogerwerf, W. A., Hellmich, H. L., Cornelissen, G., Halberg, F., Shahinian, V. B., Bostwick, J., Savidge, T. C., and Cassone, V. M. (2007) *Gastroenterology* 133, 1250-1260.
[29] Pan, X., Terada, T., Irie, M., Saito, H., and Inui, K. (2002) *Am. J. Physiol Gastrointest. Liver Physiol* 283, G57-G64.
[30] Wood, P. A., Yang, X., and Hrushesky, W. J. (2009) *Integr. Cancer Ther.* 8, 303-308.
[31] Schibler, U. and Sassone-Corsi, P. (2002) *Cell* 111, 919-922.
[32] Wang, N., Yang, G., Jia, Z., Zhang, H., Aoyagi, T., Soodvilai, S., Symons, J. D., Schnermann, J. B., Gonzalez, F. J., Litwin, S. E., and Yang, T. (2008) *Cell Metab* 8, 482-491.
[33] Rudic, R. D., McNamara, P., Curtis, A. M., Boston, R. C., Panda, S., Hogenesch, J. B., and FitzGerald, G. A. (2004) *PLoS. Biol.* 2, e377.
[34] Froy, O. (2007) *Front Neuroendocrinol.* 28, 61-71.

[35] De, G. P., Griglio, S., Pequignot-Planche, E., and Malewiak, M. I. (1977) *J. Nutr.* 107, 199-212.
[36] Wadhwa, P. S., Elson, C. E., and Pringle, D. J. (1973) *J. Nutr.* 103, 899-903.
[37] Raheja, K. L. (1973) *Comp Biochem. Physiol A Comp Physiol* 44, 1009-1014.
[38] Ahlers, I., Ahlersova, E., Smajda, B., and Sedlakova, A. (1980) *Physiol Bohemoslov.* 29, 525-533.
[39] Paulikova, E., Ahlers, I., and Praslicka, M. (1983) *Physiol Bohemoslov.* 32, 73-79.
[40] Marrino, P., Gavish, D., Shafrir, E., and Eisenberg, S. (1987) *Biochim. Biophys. Acta* 920, 277-284.
[41] Duerden, J. M. and Gibbons, G. F. (1988) *Biochem. J.* 255, 929-935.
[42] Zammit, V. A. (2000) *Biochem. Soc. Trans.* 28, 103-109.
[43] Pan, X., Zhang, Y., Wang, L., and Hussain, M. M. (2010) *Cell Metab* 12, 174-186.
[44] Hui, D. Y. and Howles, P. N. (2002) *J. Lipid Res.* 43, 2017-2030.
[45] Lowe, M. E. (1997) *Annu. Rev. Nutr.* 17, 141-158.
[46] Lowe, M. E. (2002) *J. Lipid Res.* 43, 2007-2016.
[47] Benavides, A., Siches, M., and Llobera, M. (1998) *Am. J. Physiol* 275, R811-R817.
[48] Arasaradnam, M. P., Morgan, L., Wright, J., and Gama, R. (2002) *Ann. Clin. Biochem.* 39, 136-139.
[49] Nohammer, C., Brunner, F., Wolkart, G., Staber, P. B., Steyrer, E., Gonzalez, F. J., Zechner, R., and Hoefler, G. (2003) *Lab Invest* 83, 259-269.
[50] Lichtenstein, L. and Kersten, S. (2010) *Biochim. Biophys. Acta* 1801, 415-420.
[51] Takase, S., Tanaka, K., Suruga, K., Kitagawa, M., Igarashi, M., and Goda, T. (1998) *Am. J. Physiol* 274, G626-G632.
[52] Kitazawa, M., Nagano, M., Masumoto, K. H., Shigeyoshi, Y., Natsume, T., and Hashimoto, S. (2011) *Endocrinology* 152, 2558-2567.
[53] Young, S. G., Davies, B. S., Voss, C. V., Gin, P., Weinstein, M. M., Tontonoz, P., Reue, K., Bensadoun, A., Fong, L. G., and Beigneux, A. P. (2011) *J. Lipid Res.* 52, 1869-1884.
[54] Li, C. (2006) *Curr. Opin. Lipidol.* 17, 152-156.
[55] Johansen, C. T., Kathiresan, S., and Hegele, R. A. (2011) *J. Lipid Res.* 52, 189-206.

[56] Shimba, S., Ogawa, T., Hitosugi, S., Ichihashi, Y., Nakadaira, Y., Kobayashi, M., Tezuka, M., Kosuge, Y., Ishige, K., Ito, Y., Komiyama, K., Okamatsu-Ogura, Y., Kimura, K., and Saito, M. (2011) *PLoS. One.* 6, e25231.
[57] Pan, X. and Hussain, M. M. (2012) *Biochim. Biophys. Acta* 1821, 727-735.
[58] Xiao, C. and Lewis, G. F. (2012) *Biochim. Biophys. Acta* 1821, 736-746.
[59] Abumrad, N. A. and Davidson, N. O. (2012) *Physiol Rev.* 92, 1061-1085.
[60] Hussain, M. M. (2000) *Atherosclerosis* 148, 1-15.
[61] Black, D. D. (2007) *Am. J. Physiol Gastrointest. Liver Physiol* 293, G519-G524.
[62] Hussain, M. M., Fatma, S., Pan, X., and Iqbal, J. (2005) *Curr. Opin. Lipidol.* 16, 281-285.
[63] Pan, X. and Hussain, M. M. (2007) *J. Biol. Chem.* 282, 24707-24719.
[64] Hussain, M. M., Rava, P., Pan, X., Dai, K., Dougan, S. K., Iqbal, J., Lazare, F., and Khatun, I. (2008) *Curr. Opin. Lipidol.* 19, 277-284.
[65] Fukagawa, K., Gou, H. M., Wolf, R., and Tso, P. (1994) *Am. J. Physiol* 267, R1385-R1390.
[66] Tso, P. and Liu, M. (2004) *Physiol Behav.* 83, 631-643.
[67] Martin, C., Passilly-Degrace, P., Gaillard, D., Merlin, J. F., Chevrot, M., and Besnard, P. (2011) *PLoS. One.* 6, e24014.
[68] Murai, A., Furuse, M., Kitaguchi, K., Kusumoto, K., Nakanishi, Y., Kobayashi, M., and Horio, F. (2009) *Comp Biochem. Physiol A Mol. Integr. Physiol* 154, 216-223.
[69] Diczfalusy, U., Eggertsen, G., and Alexson, S. E. (1995) *Biochim. Biophys. Acta* 1259, 313-316.
[70] Duong, H. A., Robles, M. S., Knutti, D., and Weitz, C. J. (2011) *Science* 332, 1436-1439.
[71] Schmutz, I., Ripperger, J. A., Baeriswyl-Aebischer, S., and Albrecht, U. (2010) *Genes Dev.* 24, 345-357.
[72] Schmutz, I., Albrecht, U., and Ripperger, J. A. (2012) *Mol. Cell Endocrinol.* 349, 38-44.
[73] Shelness, G. S. and Sellers, J. A. (2001) *Curr. Opin. Lipidol.* 12, 151-157.
[74] Xiao, C., Hsieh, J., Adeli, K., and Lewis, G. F. (2011) *Am. J. Physiol Endocrinol. Metab* 301, E429-E446.

[75] Sedova, L., Liska, F., Krenova, D., Kazdova, L., Tremblay, J., Krupkova, M., Corbeil, G., Hamet, P., Kren, V., and Seda, O. (2012) *Heredity (Edinb.)* 109, 63-70.

[76] Yu, H., Xia, F., Lam, K. S., Wang, Y., Bao, Y., Zhang, J., Gu, Y., Zhou, P., Lu, J., Jia, W., and Xu, A. (2011) *Clin. Chem.* 57, 691-700.

[77] Kliewer, S. A. and Mangelsdorf, D. J. (2010) *Am. J. Clin. Nutr.* 91, 254S-257S.

[78] Tong, X., Muchnik, M., Chen, Z., Patel, M., Wu, N., Joshi, S., Rui, L., Lazar, M. A., and Yin, L. (2010) *J. Biol. Chem.* 285, 36401-36409.

[79] Turek, F. W., Joshu, C., Kohsaka, A., Lin, E., Ivanova, G., McDearmon, E., Laposky, A., Losee-Olson, S., Easton, A., Jensen, D. R., Eckel, R. H., Takahashi, J. S., and Bass, J. (2005) *Science* 308, 1043-1045.

[80] Haidari, M., Leung, N., Mahbub, F., Uffelman, K. D., Kohen-Avramoglu, R., Lewis, G. F., and Adeli, K. (2002) *J. Biol. Chem.* 277, 31646-31655.

[81] Guo, Q., Avramoglu, R. K., and Adeli, K. (2005) *Metabolism* 54, 689-697.

[82] Federico, L. M., Naples, M., Taylor, D., and Adeli, K. (2006) *Diabetes* 55, 1316-1326.

[83] Pavlic, M., Xiao, C., Szeto, L., Patterson, B. W., and Lewis, G. F. (2010) *Diabetes* 59, 580-587.

[84] Wang, X. L., Zhang, L., Youker, K., Zhang, M. X., Wang, J., LeMaire, S. A., Coselli, J. S., and Shen, Y. H. (2006) *Diabetes* 55, 2301-2310.

[85] Levy, E., Spahis, S., Ziv, E., Marette, A., Elchebly, M., Lambert, M., and Delvin, E. (2006) *Diabetologia* 49, 1937-1945.

[86] Matsumoto, M., Han, S., Kitamura, T., and Accili, D. (2006) *J. Clin. Invest* 116, 2464-2472.

[87] Softic, S., Kirby, M., Berger, N. G., Shroyer, N. F., Woods, S. C., and Kohli, R. (2012) *PLoS. One.* 7, e38952.

[88] Kamagate, A., Qu, S., Perdomo, G., Su, D., Kim, D. H., Slusher, S., Meseck, M., and Dong, H. H. (2008) *J. Clin. Invest* 118, 2347-2364.

[89] Kim, D. H., Zhang, T., Ringquist, S., and Dong, H. H. (2011) *Curr. Drug Targets.* 12, 1245-1255.

[90] Wolfrum, C. and Stoffel, M. (2006) *Cell Metab* 3, 99-110.

[91] Zhang, K., Li, L., Qi, Y., Zhu, X., Gan, B., DePinho, R. A., Averitt, T., and Guo, S. (2012) *Endocrinology* 153, 631-646.

[92] Polakof, S., Medale, F., Larroquet, L., Vachot, C., Corraze, G., and Panserat, S. (2011) *J. Anim Sci.* 89, 3079-3088.

[93] Arumugam, R., Horowitz, E., Lu, D., Collier, J. J., Ronnebaum, S., Fleenor, D., and Freemark, M. (2008) *Endocrinology* 149, 5401-5414.
[94] Scarpulla, R. C. (2011) *Biochim. Biophys. Acta* 1813, 1269-1278.
[95] Zuliani, G. and Hobbs, H. H. (1994) *Hum. Mol. Genet.* 3, 215.
[96] Zvonic, S., Ptitsyn, A. A., Conrad, S. A., Scott, L. K., Floyd, Z. E., Kilroy, G., Wu, X., Goh, B. C., Mynatt, R. L., and Gimble, J. M. (2006) *Diabetes* 55, 962-970.
[97] Liu, C., Li, S., Liu, T., Borjigin, J., and Lin, J. D. (2007) *Nature* 447, 477-481.
[98] Lin, J. D., Liu, C., and Li, S. (2008) *Cell Cycle* 7, 453-457.
[99] Fernandez-Marcos, P. J. and Auwerx, J. (2011) *Am. J. Clin. Nutr.* 93, 884S-8890.
[100] Lin, J. D. (2009) *Mol. Endocrinol.* 23, 2-10.
[101] Marcheva, B., Ramsey, K. M., Buhr, E. D., Kobayashi, Y., Su, H., Ko, C. H., Ivanova, G., Omura, C., Mo, S., Vitaterna, M. H., Lopez, J. P., Philipson, L. H., Bradfield, C. A., Crosby, S. D., JeBailey, L., Wang, X., Takahashi, J. S., and Bass, J. (2010) *Nature* 466, 627-631.
[102] Duez, H. and Staels, B. (2008) *Diab. Vasc. Dis. Res.* 5, 82-88.
[103] Hylemon, P. B., Zhou, H., Pandak, W. M., Ren, S., Gil, G., and Dent, P. (2009) *J. Lipid Res.* 50, 1509-1520.
[104] Tu, H., Okamoto, A. Y., and Shan, B. (2000) *Trends Cardiovasc. Med.* 10, 30-35.
[105] Hirokane, H., Nakahara, M., Tachibana, S., Shimizu, M., and Sato, R. (2004) *J. Biol. Chem.* 279, 45685-45692.
[106] Le, M. G., Claudel, T., Gatfield, D., Schaad, O., Kornmann, B., Sasso, G. L., Moschetta, A., and Schibler, U. (2009) *PLoS. Biol.* 7, e1000181.
[107] Wooton-Kee, C. R., Coy, D. J., Athippozhy, A. T., Zhao, T., Jones, B. R., and Vore, M. (2010) *Hepatology* 51, 277-285.
[108] Lundasen, T., Galman, C., Angelin, B., and Rudling, M. (2006) *J. Intern. Med.* 260, 530-536.
[109] Shapiro, D. J. and Rodwell, V. W. (1971) *J. Biol. Chem.* 246, 3210-3216.
[110] Edwards, P. A., Muroya, H., and Gould, R. G. (1972) *J. Lipid Res.* 13, 396-401.
[111] Lavery, D. J. and Schibler, U. (1993) *Genes Dev.* 7, 1871-1884.
[112] Gielen, J., Van, C. J., Robaye, B., and Renson, J. (1975) *Eur. J. Biochem.* 55, 41-48.
[113] Kai, M., Eto, T., Kondo, K., Setoguchi, Y., Higashi, S., Maeda, Y., and Setoguchi, T. (1995) *J. Lipid Res.* 36, 367-374.

[114] Ma, K., Saha, P. K., Chan, L., and Moore, D. D. (2006) *J. Clin. Invest* 116, 1102-1109.

[115] Chiang, J. Y. (1998) *Front Biosci.* 3, d176-d193.

[116] Chiang, J. Y. (2009) *J. Lipid Res.* 50, 1955-1966.

[117] Raspe, E., Duez, H., Mansen, A., Fontaine, C., Fievet, C., Fruchart, J. C., Vennstrom, B., and Staels, B. (2002) *J. Lipid Res.* 43, 2172-2179.

[118] Mencarelli, A., Cipriani, S., Renga, B., D'Amore, C., Palladino, G., Distrutti, E., Baldelli, F., and Fiorucci, S. (2011) *Nutr. Metab Cardiovasc. Dis.*

[119] Kast, H. R., Nguyen, C. M., Sinal, C. J., Jones, S. A., Laffitte, B. A., Reue, K., Gonzalez, F. J., Willson, T. M., and Edwards, P. A. (2001) *Mol. Endocrinol.* 15, 1720-1728.

[120] Sugden, M. C., Caton, P. W., and Holness, M. J. (2010) *J. Endocrinol.* 204, 93-104.

[121] Xu, F., Gao, Z., Zhang, J., Rivera, C. A., Yin, J., Weng, J., and Ye, J. (2010) *Endocrinology* 151, 2504-2514.

[122] Xue, B. and Kahn, B. B. (2006) *J. Physiol* 574, 73-83.

[123] Um, J. H., Pendergast, J. S., Springer, D. A., Foretz, M., Viollet, B., Brown, A., Kim, M. K., Yamazaki, S., and Chung, J. H. (2011) *PLoS. One.* 6, e18450.

[124] Suter, D. M. and Schibler, U. (2009) *Science* 326, 378-379.

[125] Lamia, K. A., Sachdeva, U. M., DiTacchio, L., Williams, E. C., Alvarez, J. G., Egan, D. F., Vasquez, D. S., Juguilon, H., Panda, S., Shaw, R. J., Thompson, C. B., and Evans, R. M. (2009) *Science* 326, 437-440.

[126] Um, J. H., Yang, S., Yamazaki, S., Kang, H., Viollet, B., Foretz, M., and Chung, J. H. (2007) *J. Biol. Chem.* 282, 20794-20798.

[127] Davies, S. P., Carling, D., Munday, M. R., and Hardie, D. G. (1992) *Eur. J. Biochem.* 203, 615-623.

[128] Zhou, G., Myers, R., Li, Y., Chen, Y., Shen, X., Fenyk-Melody, J., Wu, M., Ventre, J., Doebber, T., Fujii, N., Musi, N., Hirshman, M. F., Goodyear, L. J., and Moller, D. E. (2001) *J. Clin. Invest* 108, 1167-1174.

[129] Foretz, M., Ancellin, N., Andreelli, F., Saintillan, Y., Grondin, P., Kahn, A., Thorens, B., Vaulont, S., and Viollet, B. (2005) *Diabetes* 54, 1331-1339.

[130] Lee, A. H. (2012) *Curr. Opin. Lipidol.* 23, 141-146.

[131] Lee, J. H., Giannikopoulos, P., Duncan, S. A., Wang, J., Johansen, C. T., Brown, J. D., Plutzky, J., Hegele, R. A., Glimcher, L. H., and Lee, A. H. (2011) *Nat. Med.* 17, 812-815.
[132] Takahashi, J. S., Hong, H. K., Ko, C. H., and McDearmon, E. L. (2008) *Nat. Rev. Genet.* 9, 764-775.
[133] Panda, S., Antoch, M. P., Miller, B. H., Su, A. I., Schook, A. B., Straume, M., Schultz, P. G., Kay, S. A., Takahashi, J. S., and Hogenesch, J. B. (2002) *Cell* 109, 307-320.
[134] Kako, K. and Ishida, N. (1998) *Neurosci. Res.* 31, 257-264.
[135] Reilly, D. F., Westgate, E. J., and FitzGerald, G. A. (2007) *Arterioscler. Thromb. Vasc. Biol.* 27, 1694-1705.
[136] Kino, T. and Chrousos, G. P. (2011) *Mol. Cell Endocrinol.* 336, 23-30.
[137] Hara, R., Wan, K., Wakamatsu, H., Aida, R., Moriya, T., Akiyama, M., and Shibata, S. (2001) *Genes Cells* 6, 269-278.
[138] Stephan, F. K. (1983) *Behav. Brain Res.* 7, 81-98.
[139] Stephan, F. K. (2002) *J. Biol. Rhythms* 17, 284-292.
[140] Mendoza, J. (2007) *J. Neuroendocrinol.* 19, 127-137.
[141] Stokkan, K. A., Yamazaki, S., Tei, H., Sakaki, Y., and Menaker, M. (2001) *Science* 291, 490-493.
[142] Feillet, C. A., Ripperger, J. A., Magnone, M. C., Dulloo, A., Albrecht, U., and Challet, E. (2006) *Curr. Biol.* 16, 2016-2022.
[143] Feillet, C. A., Albrecht, U., and Challet, E. (2006) *J. Physiol Paris* 100, 252-260.
[144] Levi, F. and Schibler, U. (2007) *Annu. Rev. Pharmacol. Toxicol.* 47, 593-628.
[145] Glatzle, J., Wang, Y., Adelson, D. W., Kalogeris, T. J., Zittel, T. T., Tso, P., Wei, J. Y., and Raybould, H. E. (2003) *J. Physiol* 550, 657-664.
[146] Randich, A., Tyler, W. J., Cox, J. E., Meller, S. T., Kelm, G. R., and Bharaj, S. S. (2000) *Am. J. Physiol Regul. Integr. Comp Physiol* 278, R34-R43.
[147] Zhu, J. X., Zhu, X. Y., Owyang, C., and Li, Y. (2001) *J. Physiol* 530, 431-442.
[148] Le, F. C., Irani, B. G., Magnan, C., Dunn-Meynell, A., and Levin, B. E. (2009) *Am. J. Physiol Regul. Integr. Comp Physiol* 297, R1351-R1357.
[149] Levin, B. E. (2002) *Physiol Behav.* 76, 397-401.
[150] Korn, E. D. (1966) *Science* 153, 1491-1498.
[151] Fu, J., Kim, J., Oveisi, F., Astarita, G., and Piomelli, D. (2008) *Am. J. Physiol Regul. Integr. Comp Physiol* 295, R45-R50.

[152] Fu, J., Gaetani, S., Oveisi, F., Lo, V. J., Serrano, A., Rodriguez De, F. F., Rosengarth, A., Luecke, H., Di, G. B., Tarzia, G., and Piomelli, D. (2003) *Nature* 425, 90-93.

[153] Charoensuksai, P. and Xu, W. (2010) *PPAR. Res.* 2010,.

[154] Fu, J., Dipatrizio, N. V., Guijarro, A., Schwartz, G. J., Li, X., Gaetani, S., Astarita, G., and Piomelli, D. (2011) *J. Neurosci.* 31, 5730-5736.

[155] Havel, P. J. (2001) *Exp. Biol. Med. (Maywood.)* 226, 963-977.

[156] Iqbal, J., Li, X., Chang, B. H., Chan, L., Schwartz, G. J., Chua, S. C., Jr., and Hussain, M. M. (2010) *J. Lipid Res.* 51, 1929-1942.

[157] Seugnet, L., Suzuki, Y., Thimgan, M., Donlea, J., Gimbel, S. I., Gottschalk, L., Duntley, S. P., and Shaw, P. J. (2009) *J. Neurosci.* 29, 7148-7157.

[158] Hiroyama, M., Aoyagi, T., Fujiwara, Y., Birumachi, J., Shigematsu, Y., Kiwaki, K., Tasaki, R., Endo, F., and Tanoue, A. (2007) *Mol. Endocrinol.* 21, 247-258.

[159] Kuchler, S., Perwitz, N., Schick, R. R., Klein, J., and Westphal, S. (2010) *Regul. Pept.* 164, 126-132.

[160] Kriegsfeld, L. J. and Silver, R. (2006) *Horm. Behav.* 49, 557-574.

[161] Golombek, D. A. and Rosenstein, R. E. (2010) *Physiol Rev.* 90, 1063-1102.

[162] Son, G. H., Chung, S., and Kim, K. (2011) *Front Neuroendocrinol.* 32, 451-465.

[163] Nader, N., Chrousos, G. P., and Kino, T. (2010) *Trends Endocrinol. Metab* 21, 277-286.

[164] Reddy, T. E., Pauli, F., Sprouse, R. O., Neff, N. F., Newberry, K. M., Garabedian, M. J., and Myers, R. M. (2009) *Genome Res.* 19, 2163-2171.

[165] Hanniman, E. A., Lambert, G., Inoue, Y., Gonzalez, F. J., and Sinal, C. J. (2006) *J. Lipid Res.* 47, 2503-2514.

[166] Wang, C. N., McLeod, R. S., Yao, Z., and Brindley, D. N. (1995) *Arterioscler. Thromb. Vasc. Biol.* 15, 1481-1491.

[167] Wang, C. N., Hobman, T. C., and Brindley, D. N. (1995) *J. Biol. Chem.* 270, 24924-24931.

[168] Brindley, D. N. (1995) *Int. J. Obes. Relat Metab Disord.* 19 Suppl 1, S69-S75.

[169] Li, G., Hernandez-Ono, A., Crooke, R. M., Graham, M. J., and Ginsberg, H. N. (2011) *J. Lipid Res.* 52, 971-981.

[170] Watts, L. M., Manchem, V. P., Leedom, T. A., Rivard, A. L., McKay, R. A., Bao, D., Neroladakis, T., Monia, B. P., Bodenmiller, D. M., Cao, J. X., Zhang, H. Y., Cox, A. L., Jacobs, S. J., Michael, M. D., Sloop, K. W., and Bhanot, S. (2005) *Diabetes* 54, 1846-1853.

[171] Opherk, C., Tronche, F., Kellendonk, C., Kohlmuller, D., Schulze, A., Schmid, W., and Schutz, G. (2004) *Mol. Endocrinol.* 18, 1346-1353.

In: Triglycerides
Editors: C. Araujo and D. Perez
ISBN: 978-1-62417-727-9

Chapter 3

SERUM LIPOPROTEIN LIPASE MASS AS A NOVEL BIOMARKER OF INSULIN SENSITIVITY: A ROLE IN THE EVALUATION OF LIPID- AND GLUCOSE-TARGETING DRUGS IN ADIPOCYTES AND SKELETAL MUSCLE CELLS

Masahiro Ohira[1*], Ichiro Tatsuno[1] and Kohji Shirai[2]
[1]Center for Diabetes, Endocrinology and Metabolism
[2]Department of Vascular Function, Sakura Hospital, Toho University Medical Center, Shimoshizu, Sakura-City, Chiba, Japan

ABSTRACT

Lipoprotein lipase (LPL) plays an important role in the absorption of TG from the bloodstream into the tissues. LPL abnormalities cause hypertriglyceridemia and low high-density lipoprotein (HDL)-cholesterol levels. LPL mass is usually measured after a heparin injection (postheparin LPL mass). LPL mass was found to exist in the serum

* Corresponding Author: Masahiro Ohira, MD, PhD, Center for Diabetes, Endocrinology and Metabolism, Sakura Hospital, Toho University Medical Center, 564-1 Shimoshizu, Sakura-City, Chiba, 285-0841, Japan. Tel: +81-43-462-8811; Fax: +81-43-487-4246, E-mail: 600137om@sakura.med.toho-u.ac.jp.

before heparin injection (preheparin serum). The preheparin LPL mass is not active, and the role of this serum LPL mass is not known. We sought to clarify the role of LPL. The administration of troglitazone, an insulin-sensitizer, increased the serum LPL mass, as did an insulin injection. Metabolic syndrome severity is negatively related to serum LPL mass. The homeostasis model assessment of insulin resistance (HOMA-IR) is also correlated with serum LPL mass. These data suggest that the LPL mass reflects the LPL production in the entire body and might be a good marker of insulin sensitivity.

Working from this assumption, we have assessed the effects of various lipid- and glucose-targeting drugs on LPL mass and have found several interesting results.

1) Metformin, which is mainly thought to reduce glucose synthesis in the liver, increased the serum LPL mass in type 2 diabetes mellitus patients. Thus, we observed a previously unidentified effect of metformin. In an in vitro study, metformin enhanced the LPL produced by skeletal muscle cells through the activation of adenosine monophosphate-activated protein kinase (AMPK); however, this effect was not observed in adipocytes.
2) 3-hydroxy-3-methylglutaryl coenzyme A (HMG-CoA) reductase inhibitors (statins) are widely used to reduce serum low-density lipoprotein cholesterol (LDL-C) levels. Some statins reduce serum TG levels and increase serum high-density lipoprotein cholesterol (HDL-C) levels. Pravastatin and atorvastatin increase preheparin LPL mass in patients with type 2 diabetes. Simvastatin and pitavastatin increase LPL activity in adipocytes. In skeletal muscle cells, atorvastatin and pitavastatin enhance LPL production through the activation of AMPK.

This review will define serum LPL mass and describe the effects of several lipid- and glucose-targeting drugs on serum LPL mass, in addition to discussing new mechanisms regulating triglyceride metabolism in adipocytes and skeletal muscle cells.

1. The Classical Role of Lipoprotein Lipase in Triglyceride Metabolism

Triglycerides (TG) are transported in the circulation in the form of large multi-molecular lipoprotein particles. Dietary TG and fat-soluble vitamins are packaged into chylomicrons by the intestine, while endogenously synthesized

TGs are secreted by the liver as very low-density lipoprotein (VLDL) particles. TG hydrolysis is catalyzed by lipoprotein lipase (LPL) in the blood.

LPL binds to endothelial cell-surface heparin sulfate proteoglycans [1]. LPL is not synthesized by the vascular endothelial cells but is mainly produced by adipocytes and myocytes [2]. The heart and lactating mammary gland are the other major sites of LPL synthesis [3, 4]. Lower levels of LPL are produced in macrophages, hormone-producing cells in the adrenals and ovaries, certain neuronal cells, the thoracic aorta, the spleen, the testis, the lung and the kidney [5-8]. LPL is also synthesized by hepatocytes during fetal development, but LPL production is suppressed soon after birth [9].

LPL is a TG hydrolase that is crucial for the catabolism of TG-rich VLDL and chylomicron particles [10]. This enzyme produces free fatty acids (FFAs) and monoacylglycerides, which are rapidly taken up by tissues [4]. The most important tissues in FFA metabolism are skeletal muscle, heart muscle and adipose tissue. Adipose tissue is mainly used for energy storage and supply. The FFAs in the adipose tissue are re-esterified to store energy as TG. The hydrolysis of TG by lipolytic enzymes releases FFAs into the circulation for use as an energy substrate, primarily by muscle. Monoacylglycerides are absorbed and used for gluconeogenesis in the liver. LPL deficiency or/and LPL dysfunction are known to cause severe hypertriglyceridemia.

2. The Meaning of Serum LPL Mass in Preheparin Serum (Preheparin LPL Mass)

2.1. LPL Mass in Preheparin Serum and Postheparin Serum (Postheparin LPL Mass)

Heparin releases LPL from glycosaminoglycan binding sites, as LPL binds to endothelial cell-surface heparin sulfate proteoglycans. In clinical studies, LPL levels have been analyzed using postheparin plasma [11, 12]. However, a sensitive immunoassay system using a specific monoclonal antibody against LPL has demonstrated the presence of LPL mass in preheparin serum; this LPL mass is called preheparin LPL mass [13, 14]. The activity of preheparin LPL mass is barely detectable [14]. Bezafibrate, an anti hypertriglyceridemia agent, not only increases LPL activity and mass in postheparin plasma (postheparin LPL mass) but also increases the preheparin

LPL mass [15, 16]. Thus, preheparin LPL mass is associated with postheparin LPL mass. Figure 1 shows the production and role of LPL.

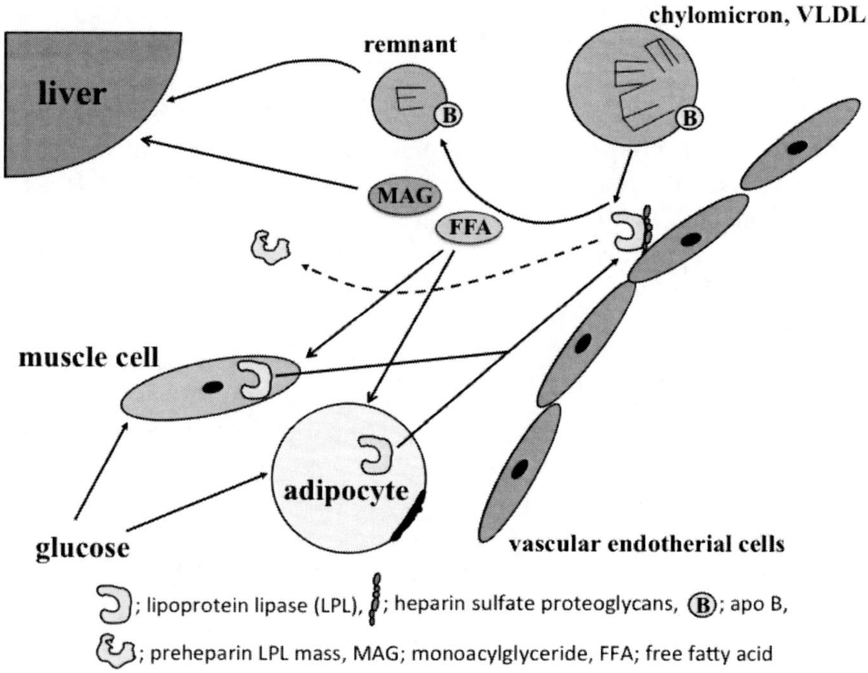

Figure 1. The production and role of lipoprotein lipase.

LPL is produced in adipocytes and skeletal muscle cells. Then, LPL is transferred to the surface of vascular endothelial cells and linked to heparin proteoglycans. LPL hydrolyzes the TGs in circulating chylomicrons and the VLDL in the blood. The LPL enzyme produces FFAs and monoacylglycerides. The liver absorbs monoacylglycerides for gluconeogenesis, the adipose tissue absorbs FFAs for energy storage and the skeletal muscle also absorbs FFAs as an energy substrate. LPL is isolated from the surface of vascular endothelial cells after hydrolyzing TG. The mass of this isolated LPL is evaluated as the LPL mass in preheparin serum (preheparin LPL mass) and is obtained from blood samples taken without a heparin injection.

2.2. The Preheparin LPL Mass Reflects LPL Production in the Entire Body and Insulin Sensitivity

The preheparin LPL mass is not affected by age or gender and does not have a circadian rhythm during the daytime [17, 18]. However, preheparin LPL mass is associated with some clinical parameters. Serum preheparin LPL mass levels correlate negatively with serum TG levels and positively with serum high-density lipoprotein cholesterol (HDL-C) levels [17]. The preheparin LPL mass also correlates negatively with fasting immunoreactive insulin (IRI) levels and the homeostasis model assessment of insulin resistance (HOMA-IR) [18, 19]. Furthermore, the preheparin LPL mass is inversely correlated with body mass index (BMI) and the intra-abdominal visceral fat area evaluated by computed tomography [20]. A low preheparin LPL mass reflects systemic oxidative stress, and preheparin LPL mass is a biomarker of metabolic syndrome severity [21]. These data indicate that preheparin LPL mass is correlated with some clinical parameters other than TG metabolism and that the preheparin LPL mass reflects the LPL production in the entire body, fat accumulation and insulin resistance. Table 1 shows the correlation between preheparin LPL mass and each clinical parameter. Some clinical studies have found different correlation coefficients because of differences in the subjects' backgrounds.

Table 1. The correlation between preheparin LPL mass and each clinical parameter

Clinical Parameter	Correlation Coefficient
Age	0.183 (18), 0.090(21)
Body Weight	-0.243(21)
Body Mass Index (BMI)	-0.046(18), -0.46(20), -0.163(21)
Systolic Blood Pressure	-0.166(18), 0.041(21)
Diastolic Blood Pressure	-0.077(18), -0.044(21)
HOMA-IR	-0.363(18), -0.272(19)
Plasma Glucose	-0.050(18), -0.294(21)
Plasma Insulin	-0.351(18)
HbAlc	-0.067(18), -0.362(21), -0.47(22)
Total Cholesterol	0.02(16), -0.095(17), 0.080(18), -0.081(21) 0.049(22), 0.03(32)
Triglyceride	-0.256(16), -0.365(17), -0.402(18), -0.48(20) -0.370(21), -0.44(22), -0.30(32)
HDL-C	0.418(16), 0.424(17), 0.471(18), 0.45(20) 0.402(21), 0.48(22), 0.19(32)
LDL-C	-0.148(17), -0.106(21), 0.15(32)
Postheparin LPL Mass	0.185(17), 0.56(22)
Adiponectin	0.562(21)
Abdominal Visceral Fat Area	-0.51(20)

HOMA-IR: homeostasis model assessment of insulin resistance,
HbA1c: glycosylated hemoglobin, HDL-C: high-density lipoprotein cholesterol, LDL-C; low-desnity lipoprotein cholesterol.

2.3. Preheparin LPL Mass is Decreased in Some Physiological States

Preheparin LPL mass is low in patients with metabolic syndrome and is also lower in type 2 diabetes patients than non-diabetic healthy subjects [21, 22, 23].

The WHO classification system classifies hyperlipoproteinemia into five different types. Type I hyperlipoproteinemia is characterized by an increase in the number of chylomicrons. Type I hyperlipoproteinemia is caused by an abnormality in either LPL or apolipoprotein C-II, which is a cofactor necessary for LPL activity. The preheparin LPL mass in patients type I hyperlipoproteinemia is very low compared with normal subjects [24, 25]. The preheparin LPL mass in patients with Type IIa hyperlipoproteinemia [total cholesterol (TC) > 220 mg/dl, TG < 150 mg/dl], is same as the preheparin LPL mass in subjects with normolipoproteinemia [17]. In contrast, the preheparin LPL mass in patients with type IIb (TC > 220 mg/dl, TG > 150 mg/dl) or type IV (TC < 220 mg/dl, TG > 150 mg/dl) hyperlipidemia is lower than the preheparin LPL mass in subjects with normolipoproteinemia [17]. The preheparin LPL mass in patients with hyperlipoproteinemia with a high TG concentration is low.

Rheumatoid arthritis (RA) is an autoimmune disease. Some clinical studies have shown that the prevalence of metabolic syndrome is increased in RA patients and that this metabolic syndrome is associated with coronary atherosclerosis and disease activity [26, 27, 28]. The preheparin LPL mass in rheumatoid patients is lower than the preheparin LPL mass in non-rheumatoid patients [29].

Pregnancy promotes insulin resistance and markedly increases plasma TG levels [30, 31]. The serum preheparin LPL mass levels in pregnant women are lower than the normal range in the first trimester and decrease further in the third trimester [32]. In the post partum period, the preheparin LPL mass recovers to within the normal range [32].

As described above, the preheparin LPL mass is decreased in various conditions that are associated with a state of insulin resistance, such as type 2 diabetes, RA and pregnancy. Table 2 shows the decrease in preheparin LPL mass in each physiological state.

Table 2. The decrease in preheparin LPL mass in each physiological state

Physiological states	Decrease in preheparin LPL mass
Metabolic Syndrome	26.3%(18), 26.9%(21)
Type 2 Diabetes	40.4%(22), 26.8%(23)
Hyperlipoproteinemia	
type I	76.4%(24), 76.9%(25)
type IIa	not decrease(17)
type IIb	29.8%(17)
type IV	22.8%(17)
Rheumatoid Arthritis	41.4%(29)
Pregnancy	
first trimester	32.8%(32)
second trimester	41.6%(32)
third trimester	52.6%(32)
post partum	not decrease(32)

2.4. Preheparin LPL Mass is Increased by Treatments for Diabetes, Hypertension or Hyperlipidemia

Preheparin LPL mass is decreased in type 2 diabetes patients [22, 23]. Insulin therapy increases preheparin LPL mass, and the preheparin LPL mass also increases when insulin therapy is switched from conventional (NPH insulin twice daily) to intensive (fast-acting insulin before every meal and one injection of NPH insulin at night) [22, 33]. Insulin increases the level of LPL mRNA in adipocytes [34].

The preheparin LPL mass is low in patients with insulin resistance [18-21]. Troglitazone, an insulin-sensitizer thiazolidinedione, increases serum preheparin LPL mass levels by 1.6 fold in type 2 diabetic patients [23]. Metformin, a biguanide class hypoglycemic agent, is widely used to reduce blood glucose levels in patients with type 2 diabetes mellitus. Metformin functions primarily by inhibiting gluconeogenesis and reducing glucose output in the liver. Metformin has other glucose lowering effects such as improving insulin resistance [35]. Metformin also increases preheparin LPL mass by 19.1% in patients with type 2 diabetes [36].

Angiotensin II receptor blockers (ARB), which are commonly used to control blood pressure, block the renin angiotensin system (RAS). Some clinical studies show that ARBs reduce the risk of developing type 2 diabetes or a new onset of diabetes [37, 38]. The adipose tissue expresses the RAS, and activation of the RAS by angiotensin II inhibits adipogenic differentiation [39, 40]. A clinical study found that circulating angiotensin II was associated with body fat accumulation and insulin resistance in obese subjects with type 2 diabetes mellitus [41]. Pioglitazone, a thiazolidinedione insulin-sensitizer, decreases circulating angiotensin II levels in type 2 diabetes patients [42]. Therefore, the RAS, especially the RAS in adipose tissue, is related to insulin resistance. Valsartan, an angiotensin type 1 receptor blocker, enhances preheparin LPL mass in type 2 diabetes patients with hypertension [43].

Table 3. The increase in preheparin LPL mass caused by each LPL-increasing therapy

Therapy	Increase in preheparin LPL mass
Insulin therapy	
insulin injection	30.1%(22)
intensive insulin therapy	19.1%(33)
(switch from conventional insulin therapy)	
Biguanide	
metformin	19.1%(36)
Thiazolidinedione (TZD)	
troglitazone	68.8%(23)
pioglitazone	16.6%(42)
Angiotensine receptor blocker (ARB)	
valsartan	14.4%(43)
Fibrate	
bezafibrate	25%(16)
Statins	
pravastatin	24.4%(44)
atorvastatin	25.3%(44)

Intensive insulin therapy; fast-acting insulin before every meal and one injection of NPH insulin at night, conventional insulin therapy; NPH insulin twice daily

Anti-hyperlipidemia agents also increase preheparin LPL mass. The preheparin LPL mass correlates with serum TG levels [17]. Bezafibrate, a drug for hypertriglyceridemia, increases preheparin LPL mass by 25% [26]. 3-hydroxy-3-methylglutaryl coenzyme A (HMG-CoA) reductase inhibitors (statins) are primarily administered to reduce serum low-density lipoprotein cholesterol (LDL-C) levels. Pravastatin increases preheparin LPL mass by 24.4%, and atorvastatin also increases preheparin LPL mass by 25.3% [44].

Preheparin LPL mass is not only increased by some insulin resistance therapies but also by hypertension or hypercholesterolemia therapies. These results indicate that changes in preheparin LPL mass are a detectable pleiotropic effect of the medication. Table 3 shows the increase in preheparin LPL mass caused by each LPL-increasing therapy.

3. The New Mechanism of LPL Production in Adipocytes and Skeletal Muscle Cells

3.1. The Mechanism by Which Metformin Enhances LPL Production

3.1.1. Metformin Reduces Serum TG Levels and Increases Preheparin LPL Mass

While metformin primarily inhibits gluconeogenesis and reduces the glucose output in the liver, this drug stimulates glucose uptake in skeletal muscle and increases fatty acid oxidation in adipose tissue [45]. This hypoglycemic agent also reduces serum triglyceride levels [46, 47]. It is thought that metformin decreases VLDL levels by reducing hepatic VLDL synthesis [45, 48, 49]. On the other hand, metformin increases LPL activity in rats and preheparin LPL mass in type 2 diabetes mellitus patients [36, 48]. The increase in LPL mass and activity might be other mechanisms by which metformin administration reduces VLDL.

3.1.2. Metformin Enhances LPL Production in Skeletal Muscle Cells but not in Adipocytes

Metformin exerts its primary effect on glucose metabolism in the liver. While LPL is mainly produced in adipocytes and skeletal muscle cells, metformin increases preheparin LPL mass in type 2 diabetes patients [2, 36]. Some studies have shown that metformin has some effects on adipocytes and skeletal muscle. For example, metformin inhibits plasminogen activator inhibitor-1 (PAI-1) in adipocytes and stimulates adenosine monophosphate-activated protein kinase (AMPK) in skeletal muscle [49, 50]. Although metformin activates AMPK in both adipocytes and skeletal muscle, metformin only promotes the induction of LPL through the activation of AMPK in skeletal muscle [51]. This result suggests that the mechanism of LPL production is different in adipocytes and skeletal muscle cells.

3.1.3. The role of AMPK and Peroxisome Proliferator-Activated Receptor (PPAR)-Γ on LPL Production in Adipocytes and Skeletal Muscle Cells

AMPK plays a key role in the regulation of glucose and lipid metabolism [52-55]. AMPK is a heterotrimeric complex consisting of a catalytic (α) subunit and two regulatory (β and γ) subunits. The N-terminus of the α-subunit contains a Thr-172 residue in the activation loop; the phosphorylation of this residue by upstream kinases is both necessary and sufficient for AMPK activation. AMPK activity is increased by muscle contraction, hypoxia, ischemia, heat shock, a decrease in pH, the inhibition of glycolysis, oxidative phosphorylation uncouplers, 5-aminoimidazole-4-carboxamide ribonucleoside (AICAR) and metformin [49, 56, 57].

In adipocytes, metformin activates AMPK but does not enhance LPL production [51]. The inhibition of AMPK by compound C, which is well known as an AMPK inhibitor, increases LPL activity in adipocytes [58]. Although metformin does not change peroxisome proliferator-activated receptor (PPAR)-γ mRNA levels and LPL mRNA levels, rosiglitazone, which is a PPAR-γ agonist, increases the levels of PPAR-γ and LPL mRNA in adipose tissue [59]. Another investigation has shown that LPL mRNA levels are highly correlated with PPAR-γ mRNA levels in white adipose tissue [60]. Thus, PPAR-γ, not AMPK, is a key mediator in enhancing LPL production in adipocytes. Therefore, metformin, an AMPK activator, does not enhance LPL production in adipocytes. In contrast, the PPAR-γ agonist pioglitazone does not increase LPL mRNA levels in skeletal muscle [60]. AMPK is a key enzyme mediating LPL production in skeletal muscle.

3.2. The Mechanism by Which Statins Enhance LPL Production

3.2.1. Statins Reduce Serum TG Levels and Increase LPL Activity or Mass

HMG-CoA reductase is a key enzyme involved in the synthesis of mevalonate from HMG-CoA. Statins, which are HMG-CoA reductase inhibitors, are widely prescribed to patients with hyperlipidemia. Statins reduce the concentration of LDL-C in the blood by enhancing LDL receptor activity [61-64]. In addition, statins also have a TG-lowering effect and a HDL-C-raising effect [65-70].

The TG-lowering effect of statins is considered to be due to reduced synthesis of VLDL in the liver [71, 72, 73]. However, some investigations have shown that TG reduction by statins is related to LPL. Simvastatin accelerates the delipidation of TG rich lipoprotein particles to increase LPL activity in type 2 diabetes patients [74]. Atorvastatin also reduces serum TG levels, and the effects of this drug are stronger than the effects of other statins, such as pravastatin, simvastatin, fluvastatin or lovastatin [75, 76]. Atorvastatin increases preheparin LPL mass and LPL activity in patients with type 2 diabetes, and these LPL changes are related to changes in TG levels [44, 77].

3.2.2. The effects of Each Statin on LPL Production in Adipocytes and Skeletal Muscle Cells

Simvastatin and pitavastatin increase LPL activity, but pravastatin and atorvastatin do not increase LPL activity in adipocytes [78]. Indeed, pitavastatin was shown to reduce serum TG levels by 22.7% in a clinical study [79]. Some investigations have shown that LPL production is enhanced by the PPAR-γ pathway in adipose tissue [59, 60]. However, the mechanism by which LPL expression is induced by pitavastatin is considered to be unrelated to PPAR-γ activation in adipocytes [78].

Both pravastatin and atorvastatin increase preheparin LPL mass in type 2 diabetes patients with hypercholesterolemia, but these drugs do not increase LPL activity in adipocytes [44, 78]. The preheparin LPL mass reflects LPL production; therefore, it is possible that pravastatin and atorvastatin increase LPL production in other LPL-producing tissues such as skeletal muscle. Atorvastatin and pitavastatin enhance LPL production, but pravastatin and simvastatin do not increase LPL production in skeletal muscle [80]. The mechanism by which these two statins and metformin enhance LPL production in skeletal muscle is the activation of AMPK [51, 80].

3.2.3. The Difference between Atorvastatin and Pitavastatin on TG Metabolism in Metabolic Syndrome Patients

Atorvastatin more effectively reduces serum LDL-C levels than pravastatin, simvastatin or lovastatin [75, 76]. Pitavastatin also reduces serum LDL levels to the same degree as atorvastatin, and some clinical studies show

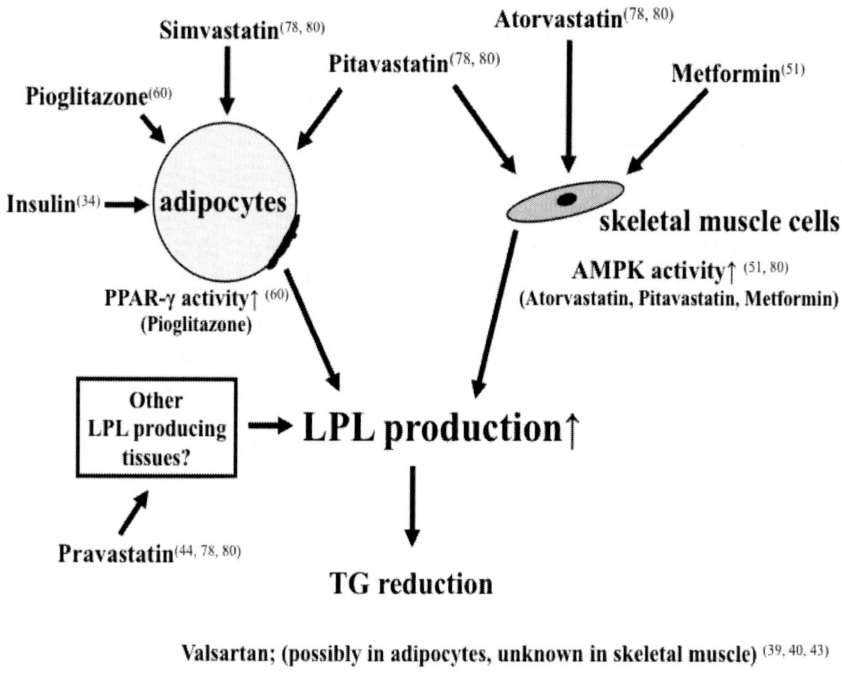

Figure 2. Drug-induced LPL production in adipocytes or skeletal muscle cells.

Simvastatin, pioglitazone and insulin enhance LPL production in adipocytes. Pioglitazone increases LPL production by activating PPAR-γ in adipocytes. Atorvastatin and metformin enhance LPL production through the activation of AMPK in skeletal muscle cells. Pitavastatin enhances LPL production in both adipocytes and skeletal muscle cells and activates AMPK in skeletal muscle. The mechanism by which pitavastatin influences LPL production in adipocytes is not related to PPAR-γ activation. Although pravastatin was shown to increase LPL mass in a clinical study, pravastatin does not enhance LPL production in both adipocytes and skeletal muscle cells. Pravastatin might enhance LPL production in other LPL-producing tissues, such as cardiac muscle cells. Therefore, the fact that adipocytes express the RAS suggests that valsartan, an angiotensin receptor blocker, could possibly enhance LPL production in adipocytes. The effect of valsartan on LPL production in skeletal muscle cells is unknown.

that atorvastatin and pitavastatin are equally effective at regulating TG metabolism [81, 82, 83). On the other hand, pitavastatin reduces the TG levels and increases the HDL-C levels of patients with metabolic syndrome significantly more than atorvastatin [83]. Furthermore, atorvastatin-mediated reductions in non-HDL-C levels are weakened with increasing body weight, waist circumference and BMI. This phenomenon is not observed with pitavastatin [81].

Non-HDL-C levels are the sum of VLDL and LDL cholesterol levels. Non-HDL-C levels are calculated routinely as total cholesterol minus HDL-C. Non-HDL-C includes all lipoproteins that contain apolipoprotein B. The differences in atorvastatin- and pitavastatin-mediated changes in non-HDL-C levels might be caused by differences in VLDL catabolism because the ability of atorvastatin or pitavastatin to reduce LDL-C levels is the same [81, 82, 83].

The varying effects of atorvastatin and pitavastatin on non-HDL-C levels appear in patients with a high body weight, large waist circumference and high BMI; these drugs also have differing effects on TG or HDL-C in patients with metabolic syndrome [83]. A high body weight, large waist circumference and high BMI usually indicate metabolic syndrome and the presence of a large amount of adipose tissue. Atorvastatin and pitavastatin enhance LPL production in skeletal muscle; however, pitavastatin, not atorvastatin, can stimulate LPL production in adipocytes [78, 80]. The difference between atorvastatin and pitavastatin on TG metabolism in patients with metabolic syndrome arises from the difference in LPL production by adipocytes. Figure 2 shows the LPL production induced by each drug in adipocytes or skeletal muscle cells.

4. The New Clinical Role of Measuring Preheparin LPL Mass

4.1. Preheparin LPL Mass is a Marker of Coronary Atherosclerosis

Preheparin LPL mass is related to glucose or lipid metabolism and is enhanced by some drugs. Controlling blood glucose or serum lipid levels prevents coronary atherosclerosis. The preheparin LPL mass is low in patients with coronary atherosclerosis or vasospasm compared with normal coronary artery subjects [84, 85]. Acute myocardial infarction (AMI) patients also show lower preheparin LPL mass than normal coronary artery subjects, and low preheparin LPL mass is a risk factor for AMI, as is hypoadiponectinemia [86, 87]. Furthermore, bear metal stent stenosis of the coronary artery is closely associated with the preheparin LPL mass concentration [88]. These results indicate that preheparin LPL mass is a marker of coronary atherosclerosis.

4.2. Preheparin LPL Mass is a Better Biomarker of Insulin Resistance than Adiponectin

Preheparin LPL mass reflects insulin resistance and is a biomarker of the severity of metabolic syndrome [18, 19, 21]. Adiponectin is also a popular biomarker of insulin resistance [89]. However, the preheparin LPL mass is a better marker of glucose metabolism, such as fasting blood glucose and glycosylated hemoglobin (HbA1c), than adiponectin [21]. LPL is primarily produced in adipocytes and skeletal muscle cells; in contrast, adiponectin is produced only in adipocytes [2, 90]. The insulin sensitizer metformin increases preheparin LPL mass but does not increase adiponectin in type 2 diabetes patients [35, 36, 91]. These results indicate that adiponectin only reflects insulin resistance in adipocytes but that preheparin LPL mass can reflect insulin resistance both in adipocytes and skeletal muscle. Preheparin LPL mass is a better biomarker of insulin resistance than adiponectin.

CONCLUSION

Based on the considerable evidence mentioned above, we feel that measuring the preheparin LPL mass provides us with useful information regarding insulin resistance and diabetes mellitus, lipid disorders and patients with a high risk of cardiovascular disease. Furthermore, preheparin LPL mass is a better biomarker of insulin resistance than adiponectin. Some medications designed to treat diabetes mellitus, hyperlipidemia or hypertension increase the preheparin LPL mass and LPL production by adipocytes and/or skeletal muscle cells. The mechanism of LPL production is different in adipocytes and skeletal muscle cells. In clinical situations, this difference influences the effects of drugs on LPL production and glucose or lipid metabolism.

REFERENCES

[1] Cheng CF, Oosta GM, Bensadoun A, Rosenberg RD. Binding of lipoprotein lipase to endothelial cells in culture. *J Biol Chem*. 1981; 256 (24): 12893-12898.

[2] Nilsson-Ehle P, Garfinkel AS, Schotz MC. Lipolytic enzymes and plasma lipoprotein metabolism. *Annu Rev Biochem*. 1980; 49: 667-693.

[3] Camps L, Reina M, Llobera M, Vilaró S, Olivecrona T. Lipoprotein lipase: cellular origin and functional distribution. *Am J Physiol*. 1990; 258 (4 Pt 1): C673-681.

[4] Braun JE, Severson DL. Regulation of the synthesis, processing and translocation of lipoprotein lipase. *Biochem J*. 1992; 287 (Pt 2): 337-347.

[5] Champs L, Reina M, Llobera M, Bengtsson-Olivecrona G, Olivecrona T, Vilaró S. Lipoprotein lipase in lungs, spleen, and liver: synthesis and distribution. *J Lipid Res*. 1991; 32 (12): 1877-1888.

[6] Goldberg IJ, Soprano DR, Wyatt ML, Vanni TM, Kirchgessner TG, Schotz MC. Localization of lipoprotein lipase mRNA in selected rat tissues. *J Lipid Res*. 1989; 30 (10): 1569-1577.

[7] Staels B, Martin G, Martinez M, Albert C, Peinado-Onsurbe J, Saladin R, Hum DW, Reina M, Vilaro S, Auwerx J. Expression and regulation of the lipoprotein lipase gene in human adrenal cortex. *J Biol Chem*. 1996; 271 (29): 17425-17432.

[8] Huey PU, Waugh KC, Etienne J, Eckel RH. Lipoprotein lipase is expressed in rat sciatic nerve and regulated in response to crush injury. *J Lipid Res*. 2002; 43 (1): 19-25.

[9] Staels B, Auwerx J. Perturbation of developmental gene expression in rat liver by fibric acid derivatives: lipoprotein lipase and alpha-fetoprotein as models. *Development*. 1992; 115 (4): 1035-1043.

[10] Bensadoun A. Lipoprotein lipase. *Annu Rev Nutr*. 1991; 11: 217-237.

[11] Saxena U, Witte LD, Goldberg IJ. Release of endothelial cell lipoprotein lipase by plasma lipoproteins and free fatty acids. *J Biol Chem*. 1989; 264 (8): 4349-4355.

[12] Peterson J, Bihain BE, Bengtsson-Olivecrona G, Deckelbaum RJ, Carpentier YA, Olivecrona T. Fatty acid control of lipoprotein lipase: a link between energy metabolism and lipid transport. *Proc Natl Acad Sci U S A*. 1990; 87 (3): 909-913.

[13] Kobayashi J, Hashimoto H, Fukamachi I, Tashiro J, Shirai K, Saito Y, Yoshida S. Lipoprotein lipase mass and activity in severe hypertriglyceridemia. *Clin Chim Acta*. 1993; 216 (1-2): 113-123.

[14] Tornvall P, Olivecrona G, Karpe F, Hamsten A, Olivecrona T. Lipoprotein lipase mass and activity in plasma and their increase after heparin are separate parameters with different relations to plasma lipoproteins. *Atherioscler Thromb Vasc Biol*. 1995; 15 (8): 1086-1093.

[15] Kobayashi J, Takahashi K, Tashiro J, Shirai K, Saito Y, Yoshida S, Hashimoto H, Fukumachi I, Niihara K, Sasaki N. Effects of treatment with bezafibrate on lipoprotein lipase activity and mass in patients with hypertriglyceridemia. *Arzneimittelforschung*. 1994; 44 (2): 145-148.

[16] Totsuka M, Miyashita Y, Ito Y, Watanabe H, Murano T, Shirai K. Enhancement of preheparin serum lipoprotein lipase mass by bezafibrate administration. *Atherosclerosis*. 2000; 153 (1): 175-179.

[17] Watanabe H, Miyashita Y, Murano T, Hiroh Y, Itoh Y, Shirai K. Preheparin serum lipoprotein lipase mass level: the effects of age, gender, and types of hyperlipidemias. *Atherosclerosis*. 1999; 145 (1): 45-50.

[18] Hanyu O, Miida T, Kosuge K, Ito T, Soda S, Hirayama S, Wardaningsih E, Fueki Y, Obayashi K, Aizawa Y. Preheparin lipoprotein lipase mass is a practical marker of insulin resistance in ambulatory type 2 diabetic patients treated with oral hypoglycemic agent. *Clin Chim Acta*. 2007; 384 (1-2). 118-123.

[19] Hanyu O, Miida T, Obayashi K, Ikarashi T, Soda S, Kaneko S, Hirayama S, Suzuki K, Nakamura Y, Yamatani K, Aizawa Y. Lipoprotein lipase (LPL) mass in preheparin serum reflects insulin sensitivity. *Atherosclerosis*. 2004; 174 (2): 385-390.

[20] Kobayashi J, Saito K, Fukamachi I, Taira K, Takahashi K, Bujo H, Saito Y. Pre-heparin plasma lipoprotein lipase mass: correlation with intra-abdominal visceral fat accumulation. *Horm Metab Res*. 2001; 33 (7): 412-426.

[21] Saiki A, Oyama T, Endo K, Ebisuno M, Ohira M, Koide N, Murano T, Miyashita Y, Shirai K. Preheparin serum lipoprotein lipase mass might be a biomarker of metabolic syndrome. *Diabetes Res Clin Pract*. 2007; 76 (1): 93-101.

[22] Miyashita Y, Shirai K, Itoh Y, Sasaki H, Totsuka M, Murano T, Watanabe H. Low lipoprotein lipase mass in preheparin serum of type 2 diabetes mellitus patients and its recovery with insulin therapy. *Diabetes Res Clin Pract*. 2002; 56 (3): 181-187.

[23] Shirai K, Itoh Y, Sasaki H, Totsuka M, Murano T, Watanabe H, Miyashita Y. The effect of insulin sensitizer, troglitazone, on lipoprotein lipase mass in preheparin serum. *Diabetes Res Clin Pract.* 1999; 46 (1): 35-41.

[24] Kern PA, Martin RA, Carty J, Goldberg IJ, Ong JM. Identification of lipoprotein lipase immunoreactive protein in pre- and postheparin plasma from normal subjects and patients with type I hyperlipoproteinemia. *J Lipid Res.* 1990; 31 (1): 17-26.

[25] Wicher I, Sattler W, Ibovnik A, Kostner GM, Zechner R, Malle E. Quantification of lipoprotein lipase (LPL) by dissociation-enhanced lanthanide fluorescence immunoassay. Comparison of immunoreactivity of LPL mass and enzyme activity of LPL. *J Immunol Methods.* 1996; 192 (1-2): 1-11.

[26] Chung CP, Oeser A, Solus JF, Avalos I, Gebretsadik T, Shintani A, Raggi P, Sokka T, Pincus T, Stein CM. Prevalence of the metabolic syndrome is increased in rheumatoid arthritis and is associated with coronary atherosclerosis. *Atherosclerosis.* 2008; 196 (2): 756-763.

[27] Zonana-Nacach A, Santana-Sahagún E, Jiménez-Balderas FJ, Camargo-Coronel A. Prevalence and factors associated with metabolic syndrome in patients with rheumatoid arthritis and systemic lupus erythematosus. *J Clin Rheumatol.* 2008; 14 (2): 74-77.

[28] de Cunha VR, Brenol CV, Brenol JC, Fuchs SC, Arlindo EM, Melo IM, Machado CA, de Castro Chaves H Jr, Xavier RM. Metabolic syndrome prevalence is increased in rheumatoid arthritis patients and is associated with disease activity. *Scand J Rheumatol.* 2012; 41 (3): 186-191.

[29] Wállberg-Jonsson S, Dahlén G, Johnson O, Olivecrona G, Rantapää-Dahlqvist S. Lipoprotein lipase in relation to inflammatory activity in rheumatoid arthritis. *J Intern Med.* 1996; 240 (6): 373-380.

[30] Jovanovic L, Pettitt DJ. Gestational diabetes mellitus. *JAMA.* 2001; 286 (20): 2516-2518.

[31] Ordovas JM, Pocovi M, Grande F. Plasma lipids and cholesterol esterification rate during pregnancy. *Obstet Gynecol.* 1984; 63 (1): 20-25.

[32] Kinoshita T, Shirai K, Itoh M. The level of pre-heparin serum lipoprotein lipase mass at different stages of pregnancy. *Clin Chim Acta.* 2003; 337 (1-2): 153-156.

[33] Miyashita Y, Ebisuno M, Ohhira M, Endoh K, Saiki A, Koide N, Ohtsuka M, Oyama T, Shirai K. Enhancement of serum lipoprotein lipase mass levels by intensive insulin therapy. *Diabetes Res Clin Pract.* 2006; 72 (1): 61-67.

[34] Raynolds MV, Awald PD, Gordon DF, Gutierrez-Hartmann A, Rule DC, Wood WM, Eckel RH. Lipoprotein lipase gene expression in rat adipocytes is regulated by isoproterenol and insulin through different mechanisms. *Mol Endocrinol*. 1990; 4 (9): 1416-1422.

[35] Bailey CJ. Biguanides and NIDDM. *Diabetes Care*. 1992; 15 (6): 755-772.

[36] Ohira M, Miyashita Y, Ebisuno M, Saiki A, Endo K, Koide N, Oyama T, Murano T, Watanabe H, Shirai K. Effect of metformin on serum lipoprotein lipase mass levels and LDL particle size in type 2 diabetes mellitus patients. *Diabetes Res Clin Pract*. 2007; 78 (1): 34-41.

[37] Dahlöf B, Devereux RB, Kjeldsen SE, Julius S, Beevers G, de Faire U, Fyhrquist F, Ibsen H, Kristiansson K, Lederballe-Pedersen O, Lindholm LH, Nieminen MS, Omvik P, Oparil S, Wedel H; LIFE Study Group. Cardiovascular morbidity and mortality in the Losartan Intervention For Endopoint reduction in hypertension study (LIFE): a randomised trial against atenolol. *Lancet*. 2002; 359 (9311): 995-1003.

[38] Julius S, Kjeldsen SE, Weber M, Brunner HR, Ekman S, Hansson L, Hua T, Laragh J, Mclnnes GT, Mitchell L, Plat F, Schork A, Smith B, Zanchetti A; VALUE trial group. Outcomes in hypertensive patients at high cardiovascular risk treated with regimens based on valsartan or amlodipine: the VALUE randomised trial. *Lancet*. 2004; 363 (9426): 2022-2031.

[39] Engeli S, Negrel R, Sharma AM. Physiology and pathophysiology of the adipose tissue renin-angiotensin system. *Hypertension*. 2000; 35 (6): 1270-1277.

[40] Saiki A, Koide N, Watanabe F, Murano T, Miyashita Y, Shirai K. Suppression of lipoprotein lipase expression in 3T3-L1 cells by inhibition of adipogenic differentiation through activation of the renin-angiotensin system. *Metabolism*. 2008; 57 (8): 1093-1100.

[41] Saiki A, Ohira M, Endo K, Koide N, Oyama T, Murano T, Watanebe H, Miyashita Y, Shirai K. Circulating angiotensin II is associated with body fat accumulation and insulin resistance in obese subjects with type 2 diabetes mellitus. *Metabolism*. 2009; 58 (5): 708-713.

[42] Saiki A, Ohira M, Endo K, Koide N, Oyama T, Murano T, Miyashita Y, Shirai K. Pioglitazone decreases plasma angiotensin II concentration in type 2 diabetes. *J Atheroscler Thromb*. 2010; 17 (6): 651-657.

[43] Saiki A, Ohira M, Endo K, Koide N, Oyama T, Murano T, Miyashita Y, Shirai K. The angiotensin II receptor antagonist valsartan enhances lipoprotein lipase mass in preheparin serum in type 2 diabetes with hypertension. *Diabetes Res Clin Pract*. 2006; 74 (3): 242-248.

[44] Endo K, Miyashita Y, Saiki A, Oyama T, Koide N, Ozaki H, Otsuka M, Ito Y, Shirai K. Atorvastatin and pravastatin elevated pre-heparin lipoprotein lipase mass of type 2 diabetes with hypercholesterolemia. *J Atheroscler Thromb*. 2004; 11 (6): 341-347.

[45] Bailey CJ, Turner RC. Metformin. *N Engl J Med.* 1996; 334 (9): 574-579.

[46] DeFronzo RA, Goodman AM. Efficacy of metformin in patients with non-insulin-dependent diabetes mellitus. The Multicenter Metformin Study Group. *N Engl J Med*. 1995; 333 (9): 541-549.

[47] Sofer E, Boaz M, Matas Z, Mashavi M, Shargorodsky M. Treatment with insulin sensitizer metformin improves arterial properties, metabolic parameters, and liver function in patients with nonalcoholic fatty liver disease: a randomized, placebo-controlled trial. *Metabolism*. 2011; 60 (9): 1278-1284.

[48] Anurag P, Anuradha CV. Metformin improves lipid metabolism and attenuates lipid peroxidation in high fructose-fed rats. *Diabetes Obes Metab*. 2002; 4 (1): 36-42.

[49] Zhou G, Myers R, Li Y, Chen Y, Shen X, Fenyk-Melody J, Wu M, Ventre J, Doebber T, Fujii N, Musi N, Hirshman MF, Goodyear LJ, Moller DE. Role of AMP-activated protein kinase in mechanism of metformin action. *J Clin Invest*. 2001; 108 (8): 1167-1174.

[50] He G, Pedersen SB, Bruun JM, Lihn AS, Richelsen B. Metformin, but not Thiazolidinediones, Inhibits Plasminogen Activator Inhibitor-1, Production in Human Adipose Tissue in Vitro. *Horm Metab Res*. 2003; 35 (1): 18-23.

[51] Ohira M, Miyashita Y, Murano T, Watanabe F, Shirai K. Metformin promotes induction of lipoprotein lipase in skeletal muscle through activation of adenosine monophosphate-activated protein kinase. *Metabolism*. 2009; 58 (10): 1408-1414.

[52] Merrill GF, Kurth EJ, Hardie DG, Winder WW. AICA riboside increases AMP-activated protein kinase, fatty acid oxidation, and glucose uptake in rat muscle. *Am J Physiol*. 1997; 273 (6 Pt 1): E1107-1112.

[53] Zheng D, MacLean PS, Pohnert SC, Knight JB, Olson AL, Winder WW, Dohm GL. Regulation of muscle GLUT-4 transcription by AMP-activated protein kinase. *J Appl Physiol*. 2001; 91(3): 1073-1083.

[54] Foretz M, Carling D, Guichard C, Ferré P, Foufelle F. AMP-activated protein kinase inhibits the glucose-activated expression of fatty acid synthase gene in rat hepatocytes. *J Biol Chem.* 1998; 273 (24): 14767-14771.

[55] Clarke PR, Hardie DG. Regulation of HMG-CoA reductase: identification of the site phosphorylated by the AMP-activated protein kinase in vitro and in intact rat liver. *EMBO J.* 1990; 9 (8): 2439-2446.

[56] Hayashi T, Hirshman MF, Fujii N, Habinowski SA, Witters LA, Godyear LJ. Metabolic stress and altered glucose transport: activation of AMP-activated protein kinase as a unifying coupling mechanism. *Diabetes.* 2000; 49 (4): 527-531.

[57] Hardie DG, Hawley SA. AMP-activated protein kinase: the energy charge hypothesis revisited. *Bioessays.* 2001; 23 (12): 1112-1119.

[58] Kim SJ, Nian C, McIntosh CH. Activation of lipoprotein lipase by glucose-dependent insulinotropic polypeptide in adipocytes. A role for a protein kinase B, LKB1, and AMP-activated protein kinase cascade. *J Biol Chem.* 2007; 282 (12): 8557-8567.

[59] Tiikkainen M, Häkkinen AM, Korsheninnikova E, Nyman T, Mäkimattila S, Yki-Järvinen H. Effects of rosiglitazone and metformin on liver fat content, hepatic insulin resistance, insulin clearance, and gene expression in adipose tissue in patients with type 2 diabetes. *Diabetes.* 2004; 53 (8): 2169-2176.

[60] Kageyama H, Hirano T, Okada K, Ebara T, Kageyama A, Murakami T, Shioda S, Adachi M. Lipoprotein lipase mRNA in white adipose tissue but not in skeletal muscle is increased by pioglitazone through PPAR-gamma. *Biochem Biophys Res Commun.* 2003; 305 (1): 22-27.

[61] The Simvastatin Pravastatin Study Group. Comparison of the efficacy, safety and tolerability of simvastatin and pravastatin for hypercholesterolemia. *Am J Cardiol.* 1993; 71 (16): 1408-1414.

[62] Illingworth DR, Tobert JA. A review of clinical trials comparing HMG-CoA reductase inhibitors. *Clin Ther.* 1994; 16 (3): 366-385.

[63] Simvastatin Pravastatin European Study Group. Comparative efficacy and tolerability of 5 and 10 mg simvastatin and 10 mg pravastatin in moderate primary hypercholesterolemia. *Cardiology.* 1994; 85 (3-4): 244-254.

[64] Weir MR, Berger ML, Weeks ML, Liss CL, Santanello NC. Comparison of the effects on quality of life and the efficacy and tolerability of lovastatin versus pravastatin. The Quality of Life Multicenter Group. *Am J Cardiol.* 1996; 77 (7): 475-479.

[65] Saito Y, Yamada N, Teramoto T, Itakura H, Hata Y, Nakaya N, Mabuchi H, Tushima M, Sasaki J, Goto Y, Ogawa N. Clinical efficacy of pitavastatin, a new 3-hydroxy-3-methylglutaryl coenzyme A reductase inhibitor, in patients with hyperlipidemia: Dose-finding study using the double-blind, three-group parallel comparison. *Arzneimittelforschung*. 2002; 52 (4): 251-255.
[66] The LIPID Study Group. Design features and baseline characteristics of the LIPID (Long-Term Intervention with Pravastatin in Ischemic Disease) Study: a randomized trial in patients with previous acute myocardial infarction and/or unstable angina pectoris. *Am J Cardiol.* 1995; 76 (7): 474- 479.
[67] Piepho RW. The pharmacokinetics and pharmacodynamics of agents proven to raise high-density lipoprotein cholesterol. *Am J Cardiol*. 2000; 86 (12A): 35 L-40 L.
[68] Ballantyne CM, Olsson AG, Cook TJ, Mercuri MF, Pederson TR, Kjekshus J. Influence of low high-density lipoprotein cholesterol and elevated triglyceride on coronary heart disease events and response to simvastatin therapy in 4S. *Circulation*. 2001; 104 (25): 3046-3051.
[69] Smilde TJ, van Wissen S, Wollersheim H, Trip MD, Kastelein JJ, Stalenhoef AF. Effect of aggressive versus conventional lipid lowering on atherosclerosis progression in familial hypercholesterolemia (ASAP): a prospective, randomized, double-blind trial. *The Lancet*. 2001; 357 (9256): 577-581.
[70] Streja L, Packard CJ, Shepherd J, Cobbe S, Ford I; WOSCOPS Group. Factors affecting low-density lipoprotein and high-density lipoprotein cholesterol response to pravastatin in the West Of Scotland Coronary Prevention Study (WOSCOPS). *Am J Cardiol*. 2002; 90 (7): 731-736.
[71] Khan BV, Fungwe TV, Wilcox HG, Heimberg M. Cholesterol is required for the secretion of the very low density lipoprotein: in vivo studies. *Biochem Biophys Acta.* 1990; 1044 (3): 297-304.
[72] Huff M, Burnett J. 3-Hydroxyl-3-methylglutaryl coenzyme A reductase inhibitors and hepatic apolipoprotein B secretion. *Curr Opin Lipidol.* 1997; 8 (3): 138-145.
[73] Yoshino G, Kazumi T, Kasama T, Iwai M, Iwatani I, Matsuba K, Matsushita M, Baba S. Effect of CS-514 (pravastatin) on VLDL-triglyceride kinetics in rats. *Atherosclerosis*. 1988; 73 (2-3): 191-195.
[74] Isley WL, Miles JM, Patterson BW, Harris WS. The effect of high-dose simvastatin on triglyceride-rich lipoprotein metabolism in patients with type 2 diabetes mellitus. *J Lipid Res*. 2006; 47 (1): 193-200.

[75] Schaefer EJ, McNamara JR, Tayler T, Daly JA, Gleason JL, Seman LJ, Ferrari A, Rubenstein JJ. Comparisons of effects of statins (atorvastatin, fluvastatin, lovastatin, pravastatin, and simvastatin) on fasting and postprandial lipoproteins in patients with coronary heart disease versus control subjects. *Am J Cardiol*. 2004; 93 (1): 31-39.

[76] Gentile S, Turco S, Guarino G, Sasso CF, Amodio M, Magliano P, Salvatore T, Corigliano G, Agrusta M, De Simone G, Gaeta I, Oliviero B, Torella R. Comparative efficacy study of atorvastatin vs. simvastatin, pravastatin, lovastatin and placebo in type 2 diabetic patients with hypercholesterolaemia. *Diabetes Obes Metab*. 2000; 2 (6): 355-362.

[77] Schneider JG, von Eynatten M, Parhofer KG, Volkmer JE, Schiekofer S, Hamann A, Nawroth PP, Dugi KA. Atorvastatin improves diabetic dyslipidemia and increases lipoprotein lipase activity in vivo. *Atherosclerosis*. 2004; 175 (2): 325-331.

[78] Saiki A, Murano T, Watanabe F, Oyama T, Miyashita Y, Shirai K. Pitavastatin enhanced lipoprotein lipase expression in 3T3-L1 preadipocytes. *J Atheroscler Thromb*. 2005; 12 (3): 163-168.

[79] Teramoto T. Pitavastatin: clinical effects from the LIVES Study. *Atheroscler Suppl*. 2001; 12 (3): 285-288.

[80] Ohira M, Endo K, Saiki A, Miyashita Y, Terai K, Murano T, Watanabe F, Tatsuno I, Shirai K. Atorvastatin and pitavastatin enhance lipoprotein lipase production in L6 skeletal muscle cells through activation of adenosine monophosphate-activated protein kinase. *Metabolism*. 2012; 61: 1452-1460.

[81] Saito Y. Pitavastatin: an overview. *Atheroscler Suppl*. 2011; 12 (3): 271-276.

[82] Chapman MJ. Pitavastatin: novel effects on lipid parameters. *Atheroscler Suppl*. 2011; 12 (3): 277-284.

[83] Yokote K, Bujo H, Hanaoka H, Shinomiya M, Mikami K, Miyashita Y, Nishikawa T, Kodama T, Tada N, Saito Y. Multicenter collaborative randomized parallel group comparative study of pitavastatin and atorvastatin in Japanese hypercholesterolemic patients: collaborative study on hypercholesterolemia drug intervention and their benefits for atherosclerosis prevention (CHIBA study). *Atherosclerosis*. 2008; 201 (2): 345-352.

[84] Hitsumoto T, Ohsawa H, Uchi T, Noike H, Kanai M, Yoshinuma M, Miyashita Y, Watanabe H, Shirai K. Preheparin serum lipoprotein lipase mass is negatively related to coronary atherosclerosis. *Atherosclerosis*. 2000; 153 (2): 391-396.

[85] Hitsumoto T, Yoshinaga K, Noike H, Kanai M, Shirai K. Clinical significance of preheparin serum lipoprotein lipase mass in coronary vasospasm. *Jpn Circ J*. 2001; 65 (6): 539-544.

[86] Hitsumoto T, Yoshinaga K, Aoyagi K, Sakurai T, Kanai M, Uchi T, Noike H, Ohsawa H, Watanabe H, Shirai K. Association between preheparin serum lipoprotein lipase mass and acute myocardial infarction in Japanese men. *J Atheroscler Thromb*. 2002; 9 (4): 163-169.

[87] Hitsumoto T, Takahashi M, Iizuka T, Shirai K. Relationship between two AMI risk factor: low serum lipoprotein lipase mass and hypoadiponectinemia. *J Atheroscler Thromb*. 2011; 18 (2): 148-156.

[88] Hitsumoto T, Takahashi M, Iizuka T, Shirai K. Relationship between preheparin lipoprotein lipase mass concentration in serum and bare metal stent stenosis. *J Cardiol*. 2006; 48 (2): 65-73.

[89] Weyer C, Funahashi T, Tanaka S, Hotta K, Matsuzawa Y, Pratley RE, Tataranni PA. Hypoadiponectinemia in obesity and type 2 diabetes: close association with insulin resistance and hyperinsulinemia. *J Clin Endocrinol Metab*. 2001; 86 (5): 1930-1935.

[90] Maeda K, Okubo K, Shimomura I, Funahashi T, Matsuzawa Y, Matsubara K. cDNA cloning and expression of a novel adipose specific collagen-like factor, apM1 (AdiPose Most abundant Gene transcript 1). *Biochem Biophys Res Commun*. 1996; 221 (2): 286-289.

[91] Phillips SA, Ciaraldi TP, Kong AP, Bandukwala R, Aroda V, Carter L, Baxi S, Mudaliar SR, Henry RR. Modulation of circulating and adipose tissue adiponectin levels by antidiabetic therapy. *Diabetes*. 2003; 52 (3): 667-674.

In: Triglycerides
Editors: C. Araujo and D. Perez
ISBN: 978-1-62417-727-9

Chapter 4

EFFECT OF PLASMA LIPIDS AND APOE GENOTYPE ON COGNITIVE DECLINE

***Fumihiko Yasuno*[1,2,*] *and Takashi Asada*[1]**

[1]Department of Neuropsychiatry, Institute of Clinical Medicine, University of Tsukuba, Tsukuba, Japan

[2]Department of Neuropsychiatry, NMU Psychiatric Institute, Nara Medical University, Nara, Japan

ABSTRACT

Although the presence of an APOE4 allele increases the risk of Alzheimer's disease (AD), there is no current evidence that the cognitive decline among those with an APOE4 allele can be prevented. Detrimental effects of APOE4 may be exacerbated by synergistic preventable risk factors, such as plasma lipids. We therefore examined the combined effect of plasma lipids and APOE genotype on cognitive function in elderly individuals. Plasma concentrations of high-density lipoprotein (HDL), low-density lipoprotein (LDL), triglyceride (TG), total cholesterol (TC), apolipoprotein E (apoE) were evaluated in 622 community-dwelling individuals aged 65 years and older. We investigated the associations between plasma lipids and cognitive function in APOE4 carrier (E4+) and APOE4 non-carrier (E4-) groups

* Fumihiko Yasuno, M.D., Ph.D., Department of Neuropsychiatry, NMU Psychiatry Institute, Nara Medical University, 840 Shijo-cho, Kashihara, Nara, 634-8522, Japan. Tel.: +81-744-22-3051; fax: +81-744-22-3854. E-mail address: yasunof@naramed-u.ac.jp

using 3-year longitudinal data. At baseline and 3 years later, cognitive scores were correlated with plasma apoE levels in both E4- and E4+, and HDL level in E4-. Our findings suggest that an interaction between apoE and HDL is affected by APOE4, and is possibly linked with a protective effect on cognitive decline in later life. Preservation of higher plasma apoE and HDL from early life is proposed as a possible strategy for maintaining cognitive function in later life, especially for APOE4-positive individuals.

Keywords: Cognitive decline, APOE genotype, Apolipoprotein E (apoE), High-density lipoprotein (HDL), Low-density lipoprotein (LDL), Triglyceride (TG), Total cholesterol (TC)

INTRODUCTION

The presence of an apolipoprotein E4 allele (APOE4) increases the risk and reduces the age at onset of Alzheimer disease (AD) in a dose-dependent manner (Rebeck et al 1993; Saunders et al 1993; Strittmatter et al 1993). Additionally, APOE4 carriers have been reported to have higher rates of cognitive decline than non-carriers before the diagnosis of mild cognitive impairment (Caselli et al 2007).

Apolipoprotein E (apoE) plays a significant role in cholesterol delivery to neurons and AD pathogenesis associated with amyloid-beta (Aβ) (Han 2010; Iurescia et al 2010; Pfrieger 2003). The plasma level of apoE has been shown to depend upon the APOE genotype (Yasuno et al, in press a,b). In elderly individuals without dementia, the interactive effect of apoE and other plasma lipids on cognitive function has also been reported to vary depending upon the APOE genotype (Yasuno et al, in press, a, b).

A complex synergism of APOE4 and cerebrovascular pathology in cognitive function of the elderly has been reported. The detrimental effect of APOE4 may be exacerbated by synergistic preventable risk factors such as plasma apoE/lipids. With stratification by APOE allele status, we examined the effect of plasma apoE/lipids on longitudinal change in the cognitive function of community-dwelling elderly using the data from a 3-year follow-up study.

METHODS

Participants

Participants were recruited in the present study from the 'Tone Project' in Tone town, Ibaraki, Japan (Miyamoto et al 2009). The sampling procedures have been described elsewhere (Yasuno et al , in press, a, b). After the assessment, a group of psychiatrists and neuropsychologists reviewed the data and reached a consensus regarding the presence or absence of psychiatric disease including dementia according to DSM-IV criteria. We excluded the data from those with history of psychiatric diseases, and 1395 volunteers participated in the first baseline study between December 2001 and April 2002. Three years later, 622 of them who had no history of stroke during follow-up could be again evaluated between December 2004 and April 2005, and we used the results of those subjects tested twice. This study uses the results of those subjects tested twice.

At the initial examination, all of the eligible subjects provided written informed consent to their participation in the study. This study was approved by the ethics committee of Tsukuba University.

Plasma Parameters

Blood samples were collected from the subjects at fasting visits at the initial examination. Plasma levels of low-density lipoprotein (LDL), high-density lipoprotein (HDL), Trigliceride (TG) and total cholesterol (TC) were measured using standard enzymatic methods on routine automated chemistry systems. Plasma apoE levels were determined by turbidimetric immunoassay. Genomic DNA was used for APOE typing. The APOE gene was amplified by the primer and amplification conditions described by Wenham and colleagues (Wenham et al 1991). After amplification, the PCR product was digested with the restriction enzyme Hha I, and subjected to electrophoresis in a 15% polyacrylamide gel.

Screening and Structured Interview

After blood sampling, all participants underwent a screening interview consisting of a structured questionnaire (questions on age, sex, education), a

15-item short version of the Geriatric Depression Scale (GDS) (Yesavage et al 1982), and evaluation of their past medical histories of cardiovascular disease, diabetes mellitus, and hyperlipidemia.

Definition of Hypertension

Prior to the baseline examination, potential participants were instructed to bring all their prescribed drugs. At the baseline examination, participants were first asked whether they had a history of treated hypertension, and then medications were checked for anti-hypertensive therapies. Baseline blood pressure was measured. Using these data, a history of hypertension requiring medication (hereafter termed HT) was defined if any one of the following conditions was present: the history of hypertension with current use of anti-hypertensive medication, or SBP/DBP$\geqq$160/100 mmHg at baseline.

Cognitive Assessment

All participants underwent the same cognitive assessment at the baseline and three-year examinations using a set of four tests to measure the following cognitive domains: attention, memory, language and reasoning. We evaluated attention by using the Japanese version of a Set-dependent activity (Sohlberg and Mateer 1986), memory ability using the Category Cued Recall test (Grober et al 1988), and language ability with a category fluency test (Solomon and Pendlebury 1998). Abstract reasoning ability was evaluated with the Similarities subtest of the Wechsler Adult Intelligence Scale-Revised (WAIS-R) (Wechsler 1981). The assessment procedures have been described elsewhere (Yasuno et al, in press a, b). A composite cognitive score was computed from the four scores using the first component of the scores of principal component analysis (Composite cognitive score=0.853*attention score + 0.809*memory score + 0.856*language score + 0.859*reasoning score).

Statistical Analysis of the Effect of Lipids/apoE

Subjects were divided into two APOE groups by E4 status with E4- (n=509) [genotypes$\varepsilon 2/\varepsilon 3$ (n=52), $\varepsilon 3/\varepsilon 3$ (n=457)] and E4+ (n=113) [genotypes ε2/ε4 (n=6), ε3/ε4 (n=99) and ε4/ε4 (n=8)] to test for the influence of genotype on the association between lipids and cognitive function.

Group differences in demographic characteristics were examined by unpaired t tests and Pearson $\chi 2$ tests. To examine the influence of group differences on cognitive function, cognitive scores were compared between groups by analysis of covariance (ANCOVA), with age, sex, years of education, GDS score, cigarette smoking and medical history of cardiovascular disease, diabetes mellitus, hyperlipidemia and hypertension as covariates. The subjects in each category were divided into three strata according to the plasma concentrations of lipids. To examine the influence of plasma lipids on cognitive function, composite cognitive scores of the three strata of plasma concentrations were compared in E4- and E4+ groups separately by ANCOVA, with age, sex, years of education, GDS score, cigarette smoking and medical history of diseases as covariates. Follow-up t tests were performed to examine differences in cognitive score among the three strata according to the levels of lipids.

Table 1. Demographic characteristics in the analysis of the effect oflipids/lipoproteins

Characteristic	ApoE4- (n =509)	ApoE4+ (n = 113)	t, χ^2 or F	p
Age, y [a]	73.0 ± 5.4	72.7 ± 4.8	t_{620}=0.5	0.6
Male, No (%) [b]	226 (44%)	43 (38%)	χ^2_1=1.5	0.2
Years of education, y [a]	10.1 ± 2.6	10.3 ± 2.9	t_{620}=0.3	0.5
GDS score [a]	2.6 ± 2.5	2.1 ± 2.2	t_{620}=1.8	0.1
Cigarette smoking, No (%) [b]	188 (37%)	37 (33%)	χ^2_1=0.7	0.4
History of disease, No (%)				
Cardiovascular disease [b]	15 (2.9%)	2 (1.7%)	χ^2_1=0.5	0.5
Diabetes mellitus [b]	20 (3.9%)	7 (6.1%)	χ^2_1=1.1	0.3
Hyperlipidemia [b]	19 (3.7%)	7 (6.1%)	χ^2_1=1.4	0.2
Hypertension [b]	195 (38.3%)	44 (38.9%)	χ^2_1=0.02	0.9
Cognitive score in 2002 [c]	42.8±11.7	40.3±11.8	$F_{1,611}$=4.1	0.04
Cognitive score in 2005 [c]	43.1±13.8	39.0±13.8	$F_{1,611}$=8.3	0.004

[a] P value was calculated by unpaired two-tailed t test.

[b] P value was calculated by Pearson χ^2 two-tailed test.

[c] P value was calculated by analysis of covariance (ANCOVA) with age, sex, and years of education, GDS score, cigarette smoking and medical history of cardiovascular disease, diabetes mellitus, hyperlipidemia and hypertension as covariates.

Data are mean±sd after adjustment for covariates.

To examine the influence of plasma lipids on change in cognitive function during the three-year follow-up, we performed repeated measures ANCOVA in the E4- and E4+ groups separately, with the level of lipids as between-subject variables, 2002 and 2005 composite cognitive scores as within-subject variables, and age, sex, years of education, GDS score, cigarette smoking and the medical history of diseases as covariates.

To examine whether the levels of lipids were related to composite cognitive scores in the E4- and E4+ groups, we performed multiple regression analysis with composite cognitive score as dependent variable and plasma lipid levels as independent variables, after adjustment for the other factors of age, sex, years of education, GDS score, cigarette smoking and medical history of diseases.

Multiple comparisons were adjusted by Bonferroni correction. All statistical tests were 2-tailed and reported at $\alpha<0.05$. Effect sizes were calculated using partial eta-squared (η^2) to estimate and compare the effect of the level of lipids on cognitive score between groups of different sample size. $\eta^2<0.01$ was regarded as no substantial effect. Statistical analysis of the data was performed using SPSS for Windows 19.0 (IBM Japan Inc., Tokyo, Japan).

RESULTS

The demographic data for the E4- and E4+ groups in the analysis of the effect of lipids/apoE on cognitive function are shown in Table 1. There were no group differences in demographic characteristics except for the cognitive score. Our finding of a higher cognitive score at 2002 and 2005 in the E4- group is consistent with previous studies (Small et al 2004).

Tables 2-3 show the median plasma concentrations of lipids for the three strata according to the tertiles of plasma levels of lipids/apoE, and the mean cognitive scores of the E4- and E4+ groups at 2002 and 2005 according to the three strata of plasma concentrations of lipids/apoE.

ANCOVA analysis evaluating the influence of lipids level on cognitive function showed a significant influence of the HDL level on composite cognitive scores at both 2002 and 2005 in the E4- group (Table 2). Subjects with higher HDL concentrations had higher cognitive scores. The effect size of the influence of the plasma HDL level on cognitive score was more than 0.01. No such significant association was observed in the E4+ group (Table 3).

Table 2. Mean cognitive test score of each tertile groups of lipid levels in ApoE4- group[a]

	Plasma lipid/apoE level, tertiles median (min-max)			ANCOVA (df=2, 498)			Group difference [b]
	Low	Middle	High	F	p	η^2	
HDL level (mg/dl)[c]	41.0 (25.0-47.0)	52.0 (48.0-60.0)	69.0 (61.0-138.0)				
Cognitive score in 2002	39.5±11.7	42.9±11.2	45.2±11.7	9.3	<0.001	0.04	A,B
Cognitive score in 2005	39.1±13.5	43.9±12.9	45.3±13.5	9.3	<0.001	0.04	A, B
apoE level (mg/dl)[d]	1.2 (0.5-1.7)	2.2 (1.8-3.0)	3.8 (3.1-10.5)				
Cognitive score in 2002	38.4±11.5	42.8±11.5	44.7±11.6	11.3	<0.001	0.04	A, B
Cognitive score in 2005	39.0±13.4	43.0±13.3	44.9±13.4	7.3	0.001	0.03	A, B
LDL level (mg/dl)[e]	73.0 (25.6-87.0)	99.0 (88.0-116.0)	134.0 (117.0-350.0)				
Cognitive score in 2002	43.1±11.8	42.9±11.7	41.7±11.9	0.7	0.5	0.003	
Cognitive score in 2005	42.9±13.6	44.1±13.4	41.6±13.7	1.4	0.2	0.006	
TG level (mg/dl)[f]	85.0 (32.0-119.0)	148.0 (120.0-183.0)	258.0 (184.0-921.0)				
Cognitive score in 2002	42.0±11.7	42.4±11.7	43.4±11.7	0.6	0.6	0.002	
Cognitive score in 2005	42.2±13.4	42.9±13.4	43.6±13.4	0.4	0.7	0.002	
TC level (mg/dl)[g]	169 (95-190)	205 (191-220)	240 (221-360)				
Cognitive score in 2002	41.2±12.0	42.3±11.7	44.2±12.0	2.5	0.1	0.01	
Cognitive score in 2005	41.2±13.8	43.0±13.4	44.4±13.8	2.2	0.1	0.009	

[a] Data are mean±SD after adjustment for age, sex, years of education, GDS score, cigarette smoking and medical history of cardiovascular disease, diabetes mellitus and hypertension. [b] Indicates significance at p< .05 after Bonferroni adjustment for multiple comparisons: A, low to middle concentration group comparison: B, low to high concentration group comparison: C, middle to high concentration group comparison. [c-g] With repeated measures ANCOVA, no significant interaction between within-subject factor of 2002/2005 cognitive scores and between-subjects factor of tertiles of plasma lipids concentration (df=2, 498, c F=1.4, p=0.3; d F=0.1, p=0.9; e F=1.5, p=0.2;f F=0.06, P=0.9; g F=0.2, p=0.8).

Table 3. Mean cognitive test score of each tertile groups of lipid levels in ApoE4+ group [a]

	Plasma lipid/apoE level, tertiles median (min-max)			ANCOVA (df=2,102)			Group difference [b]
	Low	Middle	High	F	p	η^2	
HDL level (mg/dl)[c]	41.0 (25.0-47.0)	52.0 (48.0-60.0)	69.0 (61.0-138.0)				
Cognitive score in 2002	39.8±12.5	43.3±12.8	41.6±12.7	0.7	0.5	0.01	
Cognitive score in 2005	40.0±15.8	43.2±16.1	38.7±16.0	0.7	0.5	0.01	
apoE level (mg/dl)[d]	1.2 (0.5-1.7)	2.2 (1.8-3.0)	3.8 (3.1-10.5)				
Cognitive score in 2002	40.4±12.1	33.2±12.1	50.6±12.2	7.0	0.001	0.1	B, C
Cognitive score in 2005	39.6±15.7	35.5±15.7	45.7±15.7	4.0	0.02	0.07	C
LDL level (mg/dl)[e]	73.0 (25.6-87.0)	99.0 (88.0-116.0)	134.0 (117.0-350.0)				
Cognitive score in 2002	42.6±13.0	41.0±12.6	40.8±12.9	0.2	0.8	0.004	
Cognitive score in 2005	39.0±12.1	42.1±12.0	39.7±12.3	0.4	0.7	0.007	
TG level (mg/dl)[f]	85.0 (32.0-119.0)	148.0 (120.0-183.0)	258.0 (184.0-921.0)				
Cognitive score in 2002	40.7±12.5	40.3±12.5	43.2±12.8	0.5	0.6	0.009	
Cognitive score in 2005	38.9±15.7	39.1±15.6	43.0±16.1	0.8	0.5	0.01	
TC level (mg/dl)[g]	169 (95-190)	205 (191-220)	240 (221-360)				
Cognitive score in 2002	38.8±13.3	42.4±12.6	42.0±12.8	0.7	0.5	0.01	
Cognitive score in 2005	38.3±16.8	41.5±15.9	40.4±161	0.3	0.8	0.005	

[a] Data are mean±SD after adjustment for age, sex, years of education, GDS score, and medical history of cardiovascular disease, diabetes mellitus and hypertension. [b] Indicates significance at $p < .05$ after Bonferroni adjustment for multiple comparisons: A, low to middle concentration group comparison: B, low to high concentration group comparison: C, middle to high concentration group comparison. [c-g] With repeated measures ANCOVA, no significant interaction between within-subject factor of 2002/2005 cognitive scores and between-subjects factor of tertiles of plasma lipids concentration (df=2, 102, c F=1.3, p=0.3; d F=0.04, p=1.0; e F=2.2, p=0.1;f F=0.3, p=0.7; g F=0.1, p=0.9).

A significant main effect of the apoE level was found by ANCOVA on composite cognitive scores at 2002 and 2005 in both of the E4- and E4+ group (Tables 2-3). Subjects with higher plasma apoE concentration had higher cognitive scores in both groups. The effect size of the association of the plasma apoE level on these cognitive scores was more than 0.01.

The results of ANCOVA analysis were supported by the multiple regression analysis evaluating whether the levels of HDL and apoE were related to cognitive scores. The plasma HDL level positively related to the composite cognitive score at 2002 (beta=0.13, $p<0.001$) and at 2005 (beta=0.14, $p<0.001$) in the E4- group. Plasma apoE level positively related to cognitive score at 2002 (beta=0.12, $p<0.001$) and at 2005 (beta=0.11, $p=0.001$) in the E4- group, and at 2002 (beta=0.14, $p=0.05$) and at 2005 (beta=0.13, $p=0.05$) in the E4+ group.

On the contrary, in the repeated measures ANCOVA analysis evaluating the influence of plasma lipids on the change of cognitive function during the three-year follow-up, we found no significant interaction between the concentration of lipids and the 2002 and 2005 cognitive scores in all measured comparisons (Tables 2-3).

DISCUSSION

Each of the analyses using the data from the baseline and 3-year follow-up examinations revealed that cognitive scores were associated with the plasma apoE level in both E4- and E4+, and the HDL level in E4-. We will discuss these findings.

ApoE plays a significant role in response to neuronal injury by reducing inflammation, endothelial dysfunction and lipid oxidation (Davignon et al 1999). An antioxidant role of apoE in promoting the regression of atherosclerosis has also been reported (Tangirala et al 2001). It is possible that a lower plasma apoE level impairs these normal physiological functions (Masliah et al 1995). If this is the case, a lower plasma apoE level may lead to cognitive decline and the exacerbation of cerebral degenerative changes. On the other hand, apoE is thought to bind Aβ and promote its clearance and degradation, such that a lower apoE level may reduce the efficiency of Aβ clearance, and contribute to AD pathogenesis (Stratman et al 2005).

Higher plasma levels of HDL were associated with better cognitive function in the E4- group. Low-level HDL is thought to be a risk factor for atherosclerotic diseases (Breteler et al 1994; Kalaria 2000), and it has been reported that HDL might prevent aggregation and polymerization of amyloid in the human brain (Koudinov et al 1998; Olesen and Dagø 2000). Anti-inflammatory properties of HDL could prevent inflammation from neurodegenerative processes (Cockerill et al 2001).

Recent studies have presented evidence for the involvement of internalized triglyceride-rich lipoprotein (TRL)-derived apoE in the regulation of HDL metabolism (Heeren et al 2003). The greater portion of TRL-derived apoE remains in peripheral recycling endosomes. This pool of apoE is then mobilized by HDL to be recycled back to the plasma membrane, followed by apoE re-secretion and the subsequent formation of apoE-containing HDL. This recycling of apoE may prevent cognitive decline. We found no significant association between HDL and cognitive function in the E4+ group. A recent study has shown that HDL-induced recycling of TRL-derived apoE4 is relatively inefficient (Heeren et al 2004). Thus, in the E4+ group, the inefficiency might reduce the recycling of apoE and decrease the protective effect of HDL on cognitive decline.

The present study has limitations. First, we have not quantified the longitudinal data for lipid prior to the baseline evaluation. Second, because we have no autopsies, an accurate pathological background of the cognitive decline among the E4+ carriers has not been determined. However, our longitudinal study is now continuing, and we hope that these limitations will be overcome in the future.

In conclusion, our findings suggest that a possible interaction between apoE and HDL may be linked to a protective effect on cognitive decline and that the interaction is affected by APOE4 allele in later life. It is known that neuropathological cascades leading to cognitive impairment and AD start to develop before the manifestation of cognitive impairment. Therefore, ensuring higher plasma apoE and HDL from an earlier stage of life may be useful for the maintenance of cognitive function in later life, and especially for APOE4 carriers.

ACKNOWLEDGMENT

Funding for this research was obtained from the Ministry of Health, Labor and Welfare of Japan (Grant No. H13-dementia and fracture-003).

REFERENCES

Breteler MM, van Swieten JC, Bots ML, Grobbee DE, Claus JJ, van den Hout JH, et al (1994): Cerebral white matter lesions, vascular risk factors, and cognitive function in a population-based study: the Rotterdam Study. *Neurology* 44:1246-1252.

Caselli RJ, Reiman EM, Locke DE, Hutton ML, Hentz JG, Hoffman-Snyder C, et al (2007): Cognitive domain decline in healthy apolipoprotein E epsilon4 homozygotes before the diagnosis of mild cognitive impairment. *Arch. Neurol.* 64:1306-1311.

Cockerill GW, Huehns TY, Weerasinghe A, Stocker C, Lerch PG, Miller NE, et al (2001): Elevation of plasma high-density lipoprotein concentration reduces interleukin-1-induced expression of E-selectin in an in vivo model of acute inflammation. *Circulation* 103: 108-112.

Davignon J, Cohn JS, Mabile L, Bernier L (1999): Apolipoprotein E and atherosclerosis: insight from animal and human studies. *Clin. Chim. Acta* 286:115-143.

Grober E, Buschke H, Crystal H, Bang S, Dresner R (1988): Screening for dementia by memory testing. *Neurology* 38:900-903.

Han X (2010): The pathogenic implication of abnormal interaction between apolipoprotein E isoforms, amyloid-beta peptides, and sulfatides in Alzheimer's disease. *Mol. Neurobiol.* 41:97-106.

Heeren J, Grewal T, Laatsch A, Becker N, Rinninger F, Rye K, et al (2004): Impaired recycling of apolipoprotein E4 is associated with intracellular cholesterol accumulation. *J. Biol. Chem.* 279:55483-55492.

Heeren J, Grewal T, Laatsch A, Rottke D, Rinninger F, Enrich C, et al (2003): Recycling of apoprotein E is associated with cholesterol efflux and high density lipoprotein internalization. *J. Biol. Chem.* 278:14370-14378.

Iurescia S, Fioretti D, Mangialasche F, Rinaldi M (2010): The pathological cross talk between apolipoprotein E and amyloid-beta peptide in Alzheimer's disease: emerging gene-based therapeutic approaches. *J. Alzheimers Dis.* 21:35-48.

Kalaria RN (2000): The role of cerebral ischemia in Alzheimer's disease. *Neurobiol. Aging* 21:321-330.

Koudinov AR, Berezov TT, Kumar A, Koudinova NV (1998): Alzheimer's amyloid beta interaction with normal human plasma high density lipoprotein: association with apolipoprotein and lipids. *Clin. Chim. Acta* 270:75-84.

Masliah E, Mallory M, Ge N, Alford M, Veinbergs I, Roses AD (1995): Neurodegeneration in the central nervous system of apoE-deficient mice. *Exp. Neurol.* 136:107-122.

Miyamoto M, Kodama C, Kinoshita T, Yamashita F, Hidaka S, Mizukami K, et al (2009): Dementia and mild cognitive impairment among non-responders to a community survey. *J. Cli. Neurosci.* 16:270-276.

Olesen OF, Dagø L (2000): High density lipoprotein inhibits assembly of amyloid beta-peptides into fibrils. *Biochem. Biophys. Res. Commun.* 270:62-66.

Pfrieger FW (2003): Role of cholesterol in synapse formation and function. *Biochem. Biophys. Acta* 1610:271-280.

Rebeck GW, Reiter JS, Strickland DK, Hyman BT (1993): Apolipoprotein E in sporadic Alzheimer's disease: allelic variation and receptor interactions. *Neuron* 11:575-580.

Saunders AM, Strittmatter WJ, Schmechel D, George-Hyslop PH, Pericak-Vance MA, Joo SH, et al (1993): Association of apolipoprotein E allele epsilon 4 with late-onset familial and sporadic Alzheimer's disease. *Neurology* 43:1467-1472.

Small BJ, Rosnick CB, Fratiglioni L, Bäckman L (2004): Apolipoprotein E and cognitive performance: a meta-analysis. *Psychol. Aging* 19:592-600.

Sohlberg M, Mateer CA (1986): Attention process training manual. Washington: Association for neuropsychological research and development.

Solomon PR, Pendlebury WW (1998): Recognition of Alzheimer's disease: the 7 Minute Screen. *Fam. Med.* 30:265-271.

Stratman NC, Castle CK, Taylor BM, Epps DE, Melchior GW, Carter DB (2005): Isoform-specific interactions of human apolipoprotein E to an intermediate conformation of human Alzheimer amyloid-beta peptide. *Chem. Phys. Lipids* 137:52-61.

Strittmatter WJ, Saunders AM, Schmechel D, Pericak-Vance M, Enghild J, Salvesen GS, et al (1993): Apolipoprotein E: high-avidity binding to beta-amyloid and increased frequency of type 4 allele in late-onset familial Alzheimer disease. *Proc. Natl. Acad. Sci. U. S. A.* 90:1977-1981.

Tangirala RK, Praticó D, FitzGerald GA, Chun S, Tsukamoto K, Maugeais C, et al (2001): Reduction of isoprostanes and regression of advanced atherosclerosis by apolipoprotein E. *J. Biol. Chem.* 276:261-266.

Wechsler D (1981): WAIS-R : manual : Wechsler adult intelligence scale--revised. New York: Harcourt Brace Jovanovich for Psychological Corp.

Wenham PR, Price WH, Blandell G (1991): Apolipoprotein E genotyping by one-stage PCR. *Lancet* 337:1158-1159.

Yasuno, F., Tanimukai, S., Sasaki, M., Hidaka, S., Ikejima, C., Yamashita, F., Kodama, C., Mizukami, K., Michikawa, M., Asada, T. Association Between Cognitive Function and Plasma Lipids of the Elderly After Controlling for Apolipoprotein E Genotype. *Am. J. Geriatr. Psychiatry* (in press, a). (DOI: 10.1097/JGP.0b013e318211819b).

Yasuno, F., Tanimukai, S., Sasaki, M., Ikejima, C., Yamashita, F., Kodama, C., Hidaka, S., Mizukami, K., Asada, T. Effect of plasma lipids, hypertension and APOE genotype on cognitive decline. (in press, b). (DOI: /10.1016/j.neurobiolaging.2011.12.028).

Yesavage JA, Brink TL, Rose TL, Lum O, Huang V, Adey M, et al (1982): Development and validation of a geriatric depression screening scale: a preliminary report. *J. Psychiatr. Res.* 17:37-49.

INDEX

A

B

C

D

E

F

G

H

I

J

K

L

M

N

O

P

Q

R

S

T

U

V

W